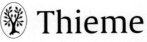

Memo

MRI Parameters and Positioning

Torsten B. Moeller, M.D.
Am Caritas-Krankenhaus
Dillingen/Saar
Germany

Emil Reif, M.D.
Am Caritas-Krankenhaus
Dillingen/Saar
Germany

With Contributions by
A. Beck
N. Bigga
Ch. Buntru
M. Forschner
B. Hasselberg
M. Hellinger
S. Köhl

S. Mattil
M. Paarmann
P. Saar-Schneider
B. Schild
K.-H. Trümmler
M. Wolff

199 Illustrations

Thieme
Stuttgart · New York

Library of Congress Cataloging-in-Publication Data

is available from the publisher.

Important Note: Medicine is an ever-changing science undergoing continual development. Research and clinical experience are continually expanding our knowledge, in particular our knowledge of proper treatment and drug therapy. Insofar as this book mentions any dosage or application, readers may rest assured that the authors, editors, and publishers have made every effort to ensure that such references are in accordance with **the state of knowledge at the time of production of the book.**

Nevertheless, this does not involve, imply, or express any guarantee or responsibility on the part of the publishers in respect of any dosage instructions and forms of applications stated in the book. **Every user is requested to examine carefully** the manufacturers' leaflets accompanying each drug and to check, if necessary in consultation with a physician or specialist, whether the dosage schedules mentioned therein or the contraindications stated by the manufacturers differ from the statements made in the present book. Such examination is particularly important with drugs that are either rarely used or have been newly released on the market. Every dosage schedule or every form of application used is entirely at the user's own risk and responsibility. The authors and publishers request every user to report to the publishers any discrepancies or inaccuracies noticed.

This book is a completely revised and enlarged new edition based on the 1st German edition published and copyrighted 2001 by Georg Thieme Verlag, Stuttgart, Germany Title of the German Edition: MRT-Einstelltechnik

Translated by Dietrich Herrmann, M.D. Hameln, Germany

© 2003 Georg Thieme Verlag, Rüdigerstraße 14, D-70469 Stuttgart, Germany
http://www.thieme.de
Thieme New York, 333 Seventh Avenue, New York, N.Y. 10001, U.S.A.
http://www.thieme.com

Typesetting by primustype R. Hurler GmbH, D-73274 Notzingen, Typeset on Textline
Printed in Germany by Druckhaus Götz, Ludwigsburg
ISBN 3-13-130581-9 (GTV)
ISBN 1-58890-149-1 (TNY)   1   2   3   4   5

Preface

Although magnetic resonance imaging, or MRI, has been with us for quite some time and is in widespread and routine use, good "recipe books" on the performance of specific actual studies are hard to find. Since all imaging modalities, and particularly MRI, are carried out by a range of operators under varying clinical circumstances, standardizing the work flow becomes ever more important, because it is only through standardization that the quality of diagnostic imaging will improve. This pared-down book attempts to close the gaps in MRI protocols for routine applications. By leaving out all extraneous information, we have put together a power-packed "how-to-do-it" book.

We have compiled protocols for most major studies, not only paying particular attention to the "classic" indications in neurology and orthopedics but also including the more recent developments such as MR angiography and MR cholangiography.

Consistent text layout is vital to clear presentation and ease of reference. The text has been structured along the same lines as the protocols themselves: starting with the preparations required for the study and the materials needed, it goes on to cover any specific points about the positioning and/or choice of coils, and then delineates the steps for each study, including not only examples of the various sequences but also available modifications. Wherever possible, we have added useful hints that may facilitate the study and point out potential complications and how to avoid them.

Experience tells us that almost every radiologist and technician has his or her own way of doing a study and prefers certain sequences and/or protocols, much as famous chefs each produce their own versions of particular dishes. Nevertheless, standardized protocols are still important and sometimes even seasoned veterans thumb through them just to check on how others have solved certain problems. We have also left plenty of space for personal notes.

This book would lose half its worth if it were based on just our own ideas about work flow. We are deeply indebted to the senior application specialists from Siemens and Philips as well as members of the sequence development units of those two companies for their commitment and innumerable valuable suggestions. Some of the work flows and choices of sequences therefore reflect the enormous expertise accumulated by these two global players in the MRI market. We are particularly grateful to Marion Hellinger, Birgit Hasselberg, Monika Forschner, and Karl-Heinz Trümmler from Siemens, and to Michael Wolff from Philips.

This resource incorporates the suggestions and expertise of many technicians in the German radiology community, and we would like to thank Andrea Beck, Silke Köhl, Pia Saar-Schneider, Sabine Mattil, Brigitte Schild, Michael Paarmann, and Dr. Christoph Buntru for their close and unwavering support.

Dillingen,   Torsten B. Möller
Fall 2002   Emil Reif

Contents

Magnetic Resonance Imaging: Spine

Magnetic Resonance Angiography

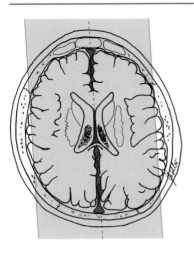

Neurocranium, sagittal, sequence 4

Tips & Tricks
— Symmetric positioning of the patient: use the bridge of the nose as reference point
— Place cushions behind the knees
— In patients with increased kyphosis, place cushions under the pelvis as well; in those with neck problems it may be necessary to raise the head somewhat and cushion it
— A mirror mounted on the head coil reduces claustrophobia

Modifications

Ruling Out Bleeding

Sequences 1 – 4 see above

Sequence 5 coronal (= orthogonal to sequence 1)
or axial (orientation as in sequence 1)

T2-weighted GRE

> **Example**
> *1.5 T:*   *1.0 T:*
> *FLASH:*   *FFE:*
> — TR = 800   — TR = 675
> — TE = 15–35   — TE = 20
> — Flip angle 20°   — Flip angle 15°
>   *0.5 T:*
>   *FFE:*
>   — TR = 900
>   — TE = 27
>   — Flip angle 15°

— Slice thickness: 5–6 mm
— Slice gap: 30% of slice thickness (≙ 1.5–1.8 mm or factor 1.3)
— Saturation slab: orthogonal to the slices (axial superior to the neck)

Neurocranium After Surgery (Tumor)

Patient Preparation
— Have an intravenous line with extension set placed

Sequences

Sequence 1 axial

T2-weighted (see basic sequence 1 above)

Sequence 2 axial

T1-weighted (see basic sequence 2 above)

Sequence 3 axial

T1-weighted (as sequence 2 but after administration of contrast agent, e.g., Gd-DTPA; activate flow compensation if needed)

Sequence 4 coronal

T1-weighted (otherwise as sequence 2 but after administration of contrast agent; activate flow compensation if needed)

Sequence 5 sagittal

T1-weighted (otherwise as sequence 2 but after administration of contrast agent; activate flow compensation if needed)

Inner Ear (e.g., Acoustic Neuroma)

Patient Preparation
— Have an intravenous line with extension set placed
Sequences
Sequence 1 coronal

FLAIR (see basic sequence 3 above)

Sequence 2 axial

T2-weighted

Example
TSE:
— TR = 4000–4500
— TE = 120–150

— Slice thickness: 3–4 mm
— Slice gap: 20 % of slice thickness (≙ 0.6–0.8 mm or factor 1.2)
— FOV: approx. 220–240 mm
— Saturation slab: parallel to the slices, 50–80 mm thick slab about 10 mm
  inferior to the most caudad slice (50–80 mm)

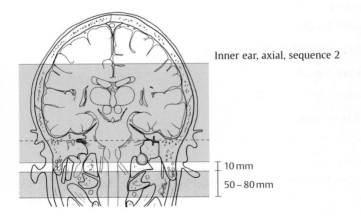

Inner ear, axial, sequence 2

10 mm
50 – 80 mm

Sequence 3 axial
(plot on coronal slice)

T1-weighted

> **Example**
> *SE:*
> — TR = 450–600
> — TE = 12–25
>   or
>
> *3-D FFE:*
> — TR = as short as possible
> — TE = 6.9 (1.5 and 1.0 T), 12–13 (0.5 T)
>   Flip angle in both cases 30°

— Slice thickness: SE (2-D) = 2–3 mm; GRE (3-D) = 0.8–1.5 mm
— Slice gap: SE (2-D) = 20% of slice thickness ($\triangleq$ 0.5 mm or factor 1.2); GRE = continuous ($\triangleq$ 0 mm or factor 1.0)
— FOV: approx. 210 mm
— Saturation slab: SE (2-D) = parallel to the slices, slab inferior to the most caudad and superior to the most cephalad slice; GRE = no saturation

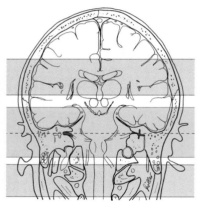

Inner ear, axial, sequence 3

Sequence 4 axial

As sequence 3, but possibly after administration of contrast agent (e.g., Gd-DTPA)

Sequence 5 axial

3-D T2-weighted, high-resolution

Example
CISS:
1.5 and 1.0 T:
— TR = 12.25
— TE = 5.9
— Flip angle 90°
— Slab thickness 30–35 mm

— No. of partitions = 40–50
— FOV = 180–200 mm (200–220 mm for 1.0 T)
1.0 and 0.5 T:
— TR = 4000
— TE = 250
— Flip angle in each case 90°

Epilepsy (Temporal Lobe Adaptation)

Sequences
— Scout: see above
— 2nd scout: sagittal across the temporal lobe

Sequence 1 axial

T2-weighted (as basic sequence 1 above)

Sequence 2 coronal

FLAIR (as basic sequence 3 above)

Sequence 3 axial (plot on scout for temporal lobe, parallel to course of temporal lobe)

T2-weighted

Example
TSE:
— TR = 3500–4500
— TE = 100–120

— Slice thickness: 3 mm
— Slice gap: 20% of slice thickness ($\triangleq$ 0.6 mm or factor 1.2)
— Matrix: 512 (256)
— Saturation slab: parallel to the slices, slab inferior to the most caudad slice

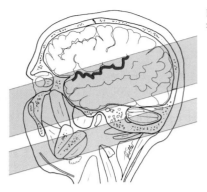

Epilepsy (temporal lobe), axial,
sequence 3

Sequence 4 coronal (orthogonal to the slices of sequence 3, across the temporal lobe, in particular its apex)

TIRM

Example	
1.5 and 1.0 T:	*0.5 T:*
— TR = 7000	— TR = 2850
— TE = 40	— TE = 20
— TI = 400	— TI = 400

— Slice thickness: 3 mm
— Slice gap: 50% of slice thickness ($\triangleq$ 1.5 mm or factor 1.5)
— Matrix: 512 (256)
— Saturation slab: no

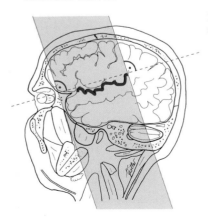

Epilepsy (temporal lobe), coronal,
sequence 4

Orbit

Patient Preparation
— Have an intravenous line with extension set placed
— Ask the patient to close his/her eyes during the study
— For women: no make-up (mascara and make-up result in artifacts); check that there is no tattooed eyeliner
— If necessary use aperture as positioning aid or for fixation on a spot
— Ask the patient to take out any contact lenses

Sequences

Sequence 1 axial

T2-weighted (as basic sequence 1 above)

Sequence 2 coronal

T2-weighted, fat-saturated

> **Example**
> *TSE, FS:*   — TR = 4000–4500
>   — TE = 90–120

— Slice thickness: 3 mm
— Slice gap: 20% of slice thickness ($\triangleq$ 0.6 mm or factor 1.2)
— FOV: approx. 200 mm
— Saturation slab: no

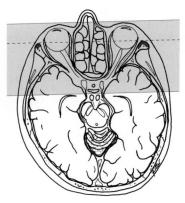

Orbit, coronal, sequence 2

Sequence 3 axial

T1-weighted, fat-saturated

Example

SE, FS:
— TR = 450–600
— TE = 12–25
  or

3-D FFE:
— TR as short as possible
— TE = 6.9 (1.0 T), 12–13 (0.5 T)
— Flip angle in each case 30°

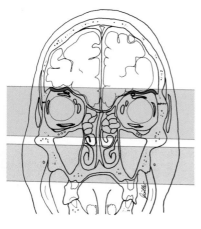

Orbit, axial, sequence 3

— Slice thickness: 3 mm (for 3-D: 1 mm)
— Slice gap: SE (2-D) = 20 % of slice thickness (≙ 0.6 mm or factor 1.2); for 3-D = continuous (0 % of slice thickness; 0 mm; factor 1.0)
— Saturation slab: parallel to the slices, slab inferior to the most caudad and superior to the most cephalad slice

Sequence 4 axial

As sequence 3, but possibly after administration of contrast agent (e.g., Gd-DTPA)

Sequence 5 parasagittal (along the optic nerve, plot on axial slice)
T1-weighted (possibly with fat saturation) after administration of contrast agent

---

Example
SE:	*3-D FFE:*
— TR = 400–600	— TR = as short as possible
— TE = 12–25	— TE = 6.9 (1.0 T), 12–13 (0.5 T)
or	— Flip angle in each case 30°

— Slice thickness: SE (2-D) = 3 mm, GRE (3-D) = 1–1.5 mm
— Slice gap: SE (2-D) = 20 % of slice thickness ($\triangleq$ 0.6 mm or factor 1.2); GRE (3-D) = continuous ($\triangleq$ 0 mm or factor 1.0)
— Saturation slab: no (but perhaps 50 % phase oversampling)

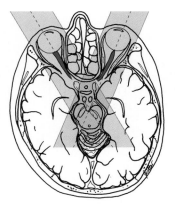

Orbit, parasagittal, sequence 5

Sella

Patient Preparation
— Have an intravenous line with extension set placed

Sequences

Sequence 1 axial

T2-weighted (as basic sequence 1 above)

Sequence 2 coronal

FLAIR (as basic sequence 3 above)

Sequence 3 coronal (plot on mediosagittal scout superior to the sella)

T1-weighted

Example	
SE:	*3-D FFE:*
— TR = 450–600	— TR = as short as possible
— TE = 12–25	— TE = 6.9 (1.0 T), 12–13 (0.5 T)
or	— Flip angle in each case 30°

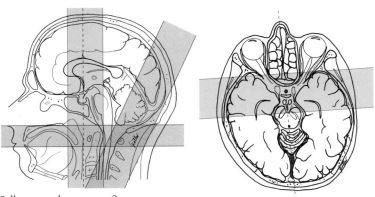

Sella, coronal, sequence 3

— Slice thickness: 2 mm (possibly 1 mm with overlap)
— Slice gap: SE (2-D) = 0–20% of slice thickness (≙ 0–0.4 mm or factor 1–1.2); GRE = contiguous (≙ 0 mm or factor 1.0)
— Saturation slab:
  • Parallel to the slices (axial superior to the head–neck junction)
  • Paracoronal posterior to the slices across the sinus
— FOV: small (e.g., 200 mm)

Sequence 4 coronal

As sequence 3, but after administration of contrast agent (e.g., Gd-DTPA)

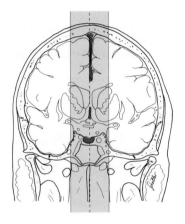

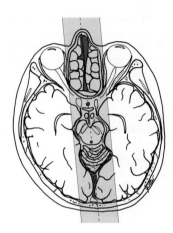

Sella, sagittal after administration of contrast agent, sequence 5

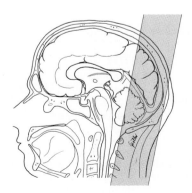

Sequence 5 sagittal after administration of contrast agent (e.g., Gd-DTPA) (plot on coronal scout superior to the sella)

T1-weighted

> **Example**
> *SE:*   *3-D FFE:*
> — TR = 450–500   — TR = as short as possible
> — TE = 12–25   — TE = 6.9 (1.0 T), 12–13 (0.5 T)
>   or   — Flip angle in each case 30°

— Slice thickness: SE (2-D) = 2 mm; GRE (3-D) = 2–3 mm, in each case with 50 % overlap ($\triangleq$ 1 and 1.5 mm respectively)
— Slice gap: SE (2-D) = 0–20 % of slice thickness ($\triangleq$ 0–0.4 mm or factor 1.0–1.2); GRE (3-D) = contiguous or overlapping
— Saturation slab: coronal slab across the posterior cranial fossa or sinus (because phase PA)
— FOV: small (e.g., 200 mm)

Technical Modification
— Possibly sequence 4 as a *dynamic* sequence

> **Example**
> — TR as short as possible   — About 15 sequences in succession
>   and turbo factor large enough
>   for the sequence to take
>   10–15 seconds

T1-weighted

> **Example**
> *TSE:*   *2-D GRE:*   *3-D FFE:*
> — TR = 450–500   — TR = 100   — TR = minimum
> — TE = 10–15   — TE minimum   — TE = 6.9 (1.0 T), 12–13
> — Turbo factor 7–12   — Flip angle: 50–60°   (0.5 T)
>   or   or   — Flip angle in each
>   case 30°

— Perhaps one noncontrast sagittal T1-weighted sequence (as sequence 5 but without contrast agent) between sequences 3 and 4
— Bolus injection (2–3 ml/s) of contrast agent at the start of sequence 1
— Dose: Gd-DTPA 0.05 mmol/kg body weight (for detection of microadenomas; „half-dosing" avoids masking of adenomas)

Soft Tissues of the Neck

Patient Preparation
— Have the patient go to the toilet before the study
— Explain the procedure to the patient
— Offer the patient ear plugs or ear protectors
— Ask the patient to undress above the waist except for underwear
— Ask the patient to remove anything containing metal (hearing aids, hair-pins, body jewelry, necklace, etc.)
— If necessary, have an intravenous line placed (e.g., if the investigation is for possible tumor)
— *Note:* Before starting the study ask the patient to swallow mostly during the pauses and to try not to swallow at all during acquisition (i.e., when the scanner is loud)

Positioning
— Supine
— Neck coil
— Cushion the legs

Sequences
— Scout: sagittal and axial (three planes are best)
Sequence 1 coronal

T2-weighted fat-saturated (plot on sagittal slice: more ventral or more dorsal depending on the purpose of the investigation; outline FOV on axial slice)

Example

TSE:
— TR = 2500–3500
— TE = 60–90
or
TIRM or STIR:
1.5 and 1.0 T:
— TR = 6500
— TE = 30–60
— TI = 140
— Flip angle 180°

1.0 and 0.5 T:
— TR = 2200–3000
— TE = 60
— TI = 140 or 100
— Flip angle 180°

— Slice thickness: 6 mm
— Slice gap: 20 % of slice thickness ($\triangleq$ 1.2 mm or factor 1.2)
— FOV: ≤ 250 mm

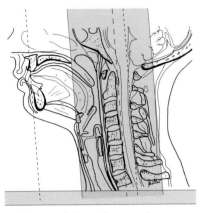 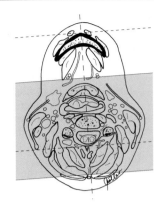

Soft tissues of the neck, coronal, sequence 1

— Saturation slab: axial below the slices for saturation of the blood vessels (if necessary with flow compensation)

Sequence 2 axial (from jugular fossa to base of skull)

T2-weighted

> **Example**
> *TSE:*
> — TR = 2500–4000
> — TE = 90–120

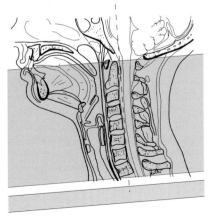

Soft tissues of the neck, axial, sequence 2

— Slice thickness: 6 mm
— Slice gap: 20% of slice thickness (≙ 1.2 mm or factor 1.2)
— FOV: approx. 180–200 mm
— Saturation slab: axial (parallel) below the slices for saturation of the vessels (if necessary with flow compensation)

Sequence 3 sagittal

T2-weighted

> **Example**
> *TSE:*
> — TR = 2500–4000
> — TE = 90–130

— Slice thickness: 6 mm
— Slice gap: 20% of slice thickness (≙ 1.2 mm or factor 1.2)
— Saturation slab: axial below the slices for saturation of the blood vessels (if necessary with flow compensation)

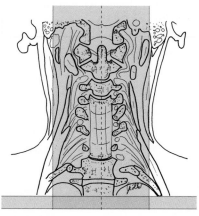 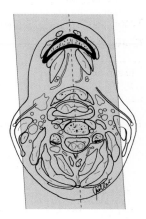

Soft tissues of the neck, sagittal, sequence 3

Sequence 4 axial

T1-weighted

> **Example**
> — TR = 450–600
> — TE = 12–25

otherwise as sequence 2

If contrast agent is administered:

Sequence 5 axial

T1-weighted (as sequence 4 but after administration of contrast agent, e.g., Gd-DTPA)

Sequence 6 coronal

T1-weighted (after administration of contrast agent)

Example
— TR = 450–600
— TE = 12–25
   otherwise as sequence 1

Tips & Tricks
— Positioning aid: center on upper border of larynx
— For really obese patients use either large flexible wraparound coil or spinal array coil (select upper section)

Chest

Patient Preparation
— Have the patient go to the toilet before the study
— Explain the procedure to the patient
— Have the patient undress except for underwear
— Ask the patient to remove anything containing metal (hearing aids, hair-pins, bra, body jewelry, necklace, etc.)

Positioning
— Supine
— Body array coil or body coil
— Cushion the legs
— If necessary, offer the patient ear protectors

Sequences
— Scout: axial and sagittal (all three planes, if possible)
Sequence 1 coronal

T2-weighted

Example

TSE, breathhold:
— TR = 3000–4000
— TE = 130–140
  or
  HASTE, breathhold:
— TR = 11.9
— TE = 95
— Flip angle 150°
  1.0 and 0.5 T:
  TSE, respiratory triggering:
— TR = 1666 or 2500 (2–3 respirations)
— TE = 100

alternatively
TSE, respiratory and cardiac triggering:
— TR = approx. 3000
— TE = 120

— Slice thickness: 8 mm
— Slice gap: 20–40% of slice thickness ($\triangleq$ 1.6–3.2 mm or factor 1.2–1.4)
— FOV: 380–400 mm
— Phase encoding gradient: LR (if at all possible have the patient raise arms above head; this may permit a smaller FOV)
— Saturation slab: no (possibly saturation slab superior to the arms)

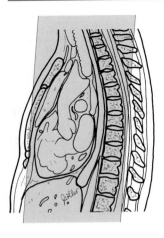

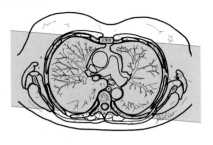

Chest, coronal, sequence 1

Sequence 2 axial

T2-weighted,
  entire lung from apex to costophrenic sinus

Example
TSE, breathhold:
— TR = 3000–4000
— TE = 130–140
— Flip angle 180°
  1.0 and 0.5 T:
  TSE, respiratory triggering:
— TR = 1666 or 2500
  (2–3 respirations)

— TE = 100
— Flip angle 90°
  or alternatively
  TSE, respiratory and cardiac trig-
  gering:
— TR = approx. 3000
— TE = 120

— Slice thickness: 8 mm
— Slice gap: 20% of slice thickness (≙ 1.6 mm or factor 1.2)
— FOV: 380–400 mm (possibly rectangular FOV)
— Saturation slab: ventral (coronal) to saturate the subcutaneous fat

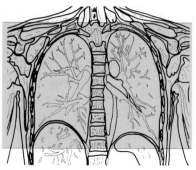 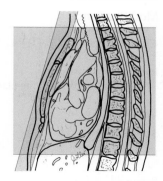

Chest, axial, sequence 2

Sequence 3 axial

T2-weighted
  otherwise as sequence 2

Example

GRE (FFE), breathhold:
1.5 and 1.0 T:
— TR = 120–140
— TE = 4–12
— Flip angle 60°

0.5 T, respiratory compensation:
— TR = 500–600
— TE = 10
— Flip angle 90°
  also perhaps (only a few slices per
  acquisition)
  1.0 and 0.5 T:
— TR = 15
— TE = 5
— Flip angle 30°

Tips & Tricks
— ECG gating possible
— For respiratory triggering ask the patient to breathe regularly
— If the investigation is for a possible tumor of the chest wall, position the
  patient on the side with the suspected tumor; this reduces motion arti-
  facts in that area

Modifications

Chest MRI with Gd-DTPA

Patient Preparation
— Have an intravenous line placed

Sequences

Sequences 1–3

(as basic sequences 1–3 above)

Sequence 4 axial

T1-weighted (as sequence 3 but after administration of Gd-DTPA) and possibly

Sequence 5 coronal

T1-weighted (as basic sequence 1 above except T1 rather than T2 but after administration of Gd-DTPA)

MRI of the Chest Wall and Mediastinum

See MRI of the Sternum (p. 25) but:
— Mark any painful area (e.g., nitroglycerin capsule)
— Adapt sequences to the purpose of the investigation, especially with regard to plotting

Sternum

Patient Preparation
— Have the patient go to the toilet before the study
— Explain the procedure to the patient
— Have the patient undress except for underwear
— Ask the patient to remove anything containing metal (hearing aids, hairpins, body jewelry, etc.)

Positioning
— Prone
— Surface coil (spine coil, flexible surface coil)
Positioning if prone position is impossible (e.g., postoperatively):
— Supine
— Body array coil or body coil, possibly large circular surface coil
— Cushion the legs
— If necessary, offer the patient ear protectors

Sequences
— Scout: axial and sagittal (all three planes, if possible)

Sequence 1 coronal across the sternum
(allow for possible oblique presentation of the chest, which will be visible in the axial image)

TIRM or STIR

Example
1.5 and 1.0 T:	*(1.5 and) 0.5 T:*
— TR = 6500	— TR = 1800
— TE = 30–60	— TE = 60
— TI = 140	— TI = 100
— Flip angle 180°	— Flip angle 90°

oder

T2-weighted, fat-saturated

Example
TSE, FS:	— TE = 100
— TR = 2000–3500	— Flip angle 90°

— Slice thickness: 2–4 mm
— Slice gap: 0–20% of slice thickness ($\triangleq$ 0–0.8 mm or factor 1.0–1.2)
— Phase encoding gradient: RL
— Saturation slab: no

Sequence 2 coronal across the sternum
(allow for possible oblique presentation of the chest)

T1-weighted

Example

— TR = 500–600	*1.0 and 0.5 T:*
— TE = 10–15	— TR = 500
— Flip angle 90°	— TE = 10–20
	— Flip angle 90°

— Slice thickness: 2–4 mm
— Slice gap: 0–20% of slice thickness ($\triangleq$ 0–0.8 mm or factor 1.0–1.2)
— Phase encoding gradient: RL
— Saturation slab: no

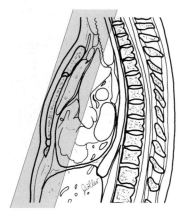
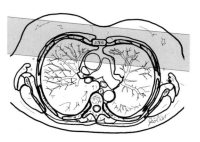

Sternum, coronal,
sequences 1 and 2

Sequence 3 axial

T2-weighted entire sternum from the jugular fossa to the xiphoid process, or, in the case of investigation for pathologic findings of the sterno-clavicular joints, across the sternoclavicular joints

---

Example

1.5 and 1.0 T:	*(1.0 and) 0.5 T:*
TSE, breathhold:	*TSE, respiratory triggering:*
— TR = 3000–4000	— TR = 1666 or 2500 (2–3 respira-
— TE = 130–140	tions)
— Flip angle 180°	— TE = 100
	— Flip angle 90°

- — Slice thickness: 4–6 mm
- — Slice gap: 20% of slice thickness ($\triangleq$ 0.8–1.2 mm or factor 1.2)
- — Phase encoding gradient: RL
- — Saturation slab: no

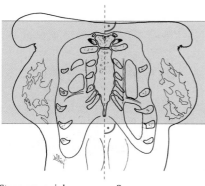
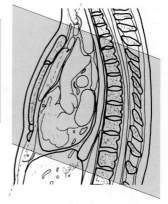

Sternum, axial, sequence 3

Sequence 4 sagittal across the sternum
(allow for possible oblique presentation of the chest)

T1-weighted

Example
- — TR = 450–600
- — TE = 10–20
- — Flip angle 90°

---

or

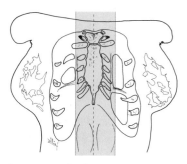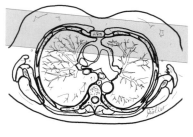

Sternum, sagittal, sequence 4

T2-weighted

> **Example**
>
> | | |
> |---|---|
> | *1.5 and 1.0 T:* | *1.0 and 0.5 T:* |
> | *TSE, breathhold:* | *TSE, respiratory triggering:* |
> | — TR = 3000–4000 | — TR = 1666 or 2500 (2–3 respira- |
> | — TE = 130–140 | tions) |
> | — Flip angle 180° | — TE = 100 |
> | | — Flip angle 90° |

- Slice thickness: 4 mm
- Slice gap: 20% of slice thickness (≙ 0.8 mm or factor 1.2)
- Phase encoding gradient: HF
- Saturation slab: no (but with phase oversampling)

> **Tips & Tricks**
> - ECG gating possible
> - For respiratory triggering ask the patient to breathe regularly

Modifications

Contrast MRI of the Sternum

Patient Preparation
- Have an intravenous line placed

Sequences

Sequences 1–3

(as basic sequences 1–3 above)

Sequence 4

T1-weighted coronal
(as basic sequence 2 above, but after administration of Gd-DTPA) and possibly

Sequence 5

T1-weighted axial
(as sequence 3, but after administration of Gd-DTPA)

Breast

Patient Preparation
— Have the patient go to the toilet before the study
— Explain the procedure to the patient
— Offer the patient ear protectors or ear plugs
— Have the patient undress completely above the waist
— Ask the patient to remove anything containing metal (hearing aids, hair-pins, body jewelry, necklace, etc.)
— Have an intravenous line placed

Positioning
— Prone
— Breast coil
— Arms alongside the body or in front of the head, forehead resting on the hands

Sequences
— Scout: axial, coronal, and parasagittal

Sequence 1 axial

T2-weighted

Example
TSE:
— TR = 3000–5000
— TE = 100–120

— Slice thickness: 4 mm
— Slice gap: 0–20% of slice thickness ($\triangleq$ 0–0.8 mm or factor 1.0–1.2)
— Phase encoding gradient: LR (because of cardiac motion)
— Saturation slab: no

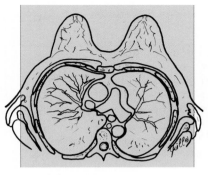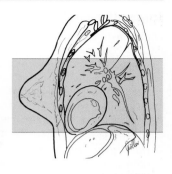

Breast, axial, sequence 1

Sequence 2 axial

T2-weighted 3-D GRE

Example

1.5 T:
FFE:
— TR = 11
— TE = 4.6
— Flip angle 25°
1.0 T:
— TR = 8.5–12
— TE = 5.3–6.1
— Flip angle 20–25°

0.5 T:
— TR = 7.7–10
— TE = 2.5–3
— Flip angle 25°
or
— TR = 24
— TE = 13
— Flip angle 50°

— Slab thickness: 128 mm
— No. of partitions: 32
— (Effective) slice thickness: < 4 mm
— FOV: 30–35 mm
— Phase encoding gradient: LR
— Saturation slab: no

Sequences 3–8

T1-weighted axial as sequence 2 but after administration of contrast agent (Gd-DTPA 0.1 mmol/kg body weight), no delay between the sequences (sequence duration 50–90 seconds), and possibly coronal images

Sequence 9 coronal

T1-weighted 3-D GRE

> **Example**
> — TR = 8–12
> — TE = 4.5–6
> — Flip angle 20–25°

— Slab thickness: 128 mm
— No. of partitions: 32
— (Effective) slice thickness: < 4 mm
— FOV: 30–35 mm
— Phase encoding gradient: cephalocaudal
— Saturation slab: no

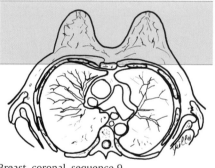 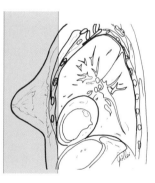

Breast, coronal, sequence 9

Postprocessing
— Subtract sequence 2 from, e.g., sequence 4
— Dynamic assessment of pathologic contrast enhancements

> **Tips & Tricks**
> — For a small breast, cushion the inside of the coil with some padding (reduces motion artifacts)
> — A tight-fitting T-shirt can also be quite effective in immobilizing the breasts

Magnetic Resonance Imaging:
Abdomen, Pelvis

Upper Abdomen/Liver

Patient Preparation
— Have the patient go to the toilet before the study
— Explain the procedure to the patient
— Ask the patient to undress except for underwear
— Ask the patient to remove anything containing metal (hearing aids, hairpins, body jewelry, etc.)
— Depending on the purpose of the investigation, have the patient drink a contrast solution (e.g., Lumirem, Guerbet S.A., France) 30 minutes before the beginning of the study

Positioning
— Supine
— Body array coil or body coil
— Cushion the legs
— If necessary offer the patient ear protectors
— If necessary have the patient raise his/her arms above his/her head

Sequences
— Scout: coronal and sagittal (three planes, if possible)

Sequence 1 axial

T2-weighted from the dome of the liver to the aortic bifurcation

---

Example

TSE, breathhold: *1.0 and 0.5 T:*
  — TR = 3000–4000   *TSE, respiratory triggering:*
  — TE = 100–140   — TR = 1666 or 2500 (2–3 respira-
or   tions)
HASTE, breathhold: — TE = 100
  — TR = 11.9
  — TE = 95
  — Flip angle 150°

— Slice thickness: 8 mm
— Slice gap: 10–20% of slice thickness ($\triangleq$ 0.8–1.6 mm or factor 1.1–1.2)
— FOV: 360–400 mm (possibly rectangular FOV)
— Saturation slab: axial (parallel) superior to the slices for saturation of the vessels and ventral (coronal) for saturation of the subcutaneous fat

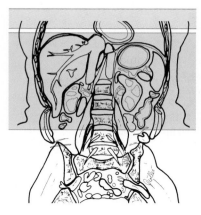

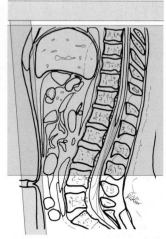

Liver/upper abdomen, axial,
sequence 1

Sequence 2 axial

T1-weighted, otherwise as sequence 1

Example
1.5 and 1.0 T:
GRE (FLASH), breathhold:
— TR = 120–140
— TE = 4
— Flip angle 60°
or

1.0 T:
TSE, breathhold:
— TR = 300
— TE = 12; repeat 3 or 4 times until
  the complete organ has been im-
  aged
0.5 T:
SE, respiratory compensation:
— TR = 500–600
— TE = 10–20
— Flip angle 90°

Sequence 3 coronal

T2-weighted

> **Example**
> *1.5 and 1.0 T:* *1.0 and 0.5 T:*
> *TSE, breathhold:* *TSE, respiratory triggering:*
> — TR = 3000–4000 — TR = 1900–2300
> — TE = 90–140 — TE = 100
> — Flip angle 180° — Flip angle 90°

or

HASTE, breathhold

> **Example**
> — TR = 11.9
> — TE = 95
> — Flip angle 150°

— Slice thickness: 8 mm
— Slice gap: 0 (3-D) – 20 % (TSE) of slice thickness ($\triangleq$ 0–1.6 mm or factor 1.0–1.2)
— FOV: 380–400 mm
— Saturation slab: axial superior to the slices for saturation of the blood vessels

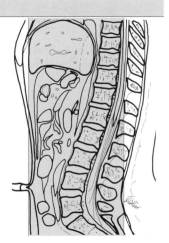
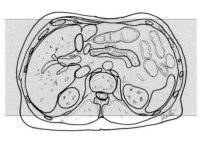

Liver/upper abdomen, coronal, sequence 3

Tips & Tricks
— Hyoscine butylbromide can be given intravenously to attenuate intestinal motility
— Oral contrast agent is given for intestinal contrast
— When imaging the biliary tree, use single-slice technique to set up the longer multislice sequences

Modifications

Liver MRI with Superparamagnetic Contrast Agent

Sequences

Sequence 1 axial

(as basic sequence 1)

Sequence 2 axial

T1-weighted (otherwise as basic sequence 1)
Move patient out of the scanner; infuse the intravenous contrast agent (Feridex I.V., Guerbet S.A., France)

Approx. 1–1.5 hours after the infusion has been started:

Sequence 3 axial

T2-weighted (as above, but after administration of contrast agent)

Sequence 4 axial

T1-weighted (as above, but after administration of contrast agent)

Sequence 5 coronal

T2-weighted (as above, but after administration of contrast agent)

MRI of the Liver with Gd-DTPA

Patient Preparation
— Have an intravenous line placed

Sequences

Sequence 1 axial

T2-weighted (as basic sequence 1)

Sequence 2 axial

T1-weighted (as basic sequence 1)

Sequence 3 axial

T1-weighted (as above, but after administration of Gd-DTPA) and possibly

Sequences 3–8 axial

T1-weighted (dynamic; sequences in immediate succession with pauses for breath between) and possibly

Sequence 9 axial

T1-weighted (as delayed image about 5 minutes after the infusion)

Biliary Tree

Sequence

Paracoronal sequence (adjusted to the course of the common bile duct = about 0–30° off the horizontal plane, plot on axial image)

Single-slice technique: T2-weighted, fat-saturated, long TE, large turbo factor

---

Example

1.5 and 1.0 T:
— TR = 2800
— TE = 1100
— Flip angle 150°
— Slice thickness = 70 mm

(1.0 and) 0.5 T:
2-D TSE, FS (SPIR):
— TR = 8000
— TE = 1250
— Flip angle 90°
No MIP analysis required

---

and/or

T2-weighted, fat-saturated

Example

1.5 T:
HASTE:
— TR = 11.9
— TE = 95
— Flip angle 150°
1.0 T:
TSE, respiratory triggering:
— TR = 5000
— TE = 250
— Matrix = 192 × 256

— Slice thickness = 3.5 mm, possibly with 50% overlap, 30 slices
0.5 T:
3-D IR-TSE, respiratory triggering:
— TR = 1666 or 2500
— TE = 700
— TI = 90
— Slice thickness 4 mm with 50% overlap = 2 mm, with subsequent MIP analysis

---

— FOV: large (at least 35 cm in order to avoid foldover)

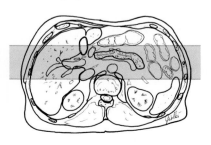

Biliary tree (para-)coronal

Small Intestine (Hydro-MRI)

Patient Preparation
— The patient should fast for at least four hours before the study (fluids are permitted)
— One hour before the study begins, the patient should drink 1000 ml of a 2.5% mannitol solution
— Have the patient go to the toilet before the study
— Explain the procedure to the patient
— Ask the patient to undress except for underwear
— Ask the patient to remove anything containing metal (hearing aids, hair-pins, body jewelry, etc.)
— Have an intravenous line placed

Positioning
— Supine
— Body array coil or body coil
— Cushion the legs
— If necessary, offer the patient ear protectors
— If necessary, have the patient raise his/her arms over his/her head

Sequences
— Scout: coronal and sagittal (three planes, if possible); injection of hyoscine butylbromide 20 mg

Sequence 1 axial

T2-weighted from dome of liver to pelvic outlet, fat-saturated

Example
1.5 and 1.0 T: *HASTE sequence, breathhold:*
TSE, FS, breathhold: — TR = 11.9
— TR = 3000–4000   — TE = 95
— TE = 100–140   — Flip angle 150°
(1.0 and) 0.5 T:
TSE, FS, respiratory triggering:
— TR = 1666 or 2500 (2–3 respirations)
— TE = 100
or

— Slice thickness: 8 mm
— Slice gap: 20% of slice thickness (≙ 1.6 mm or factor 1.2)
— FOV: large (at least 35 cm in order to avoid foldover), about 450 mm
— Saturation slab: axial superior to the slices for saturation of the vessels
  and ventral (coronal) for saturation of the subcutaneous fat
  and possibly

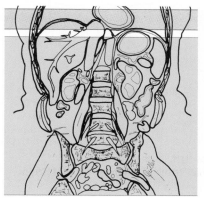
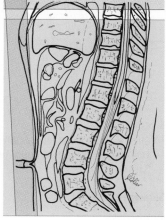

Small intestine (hydro-MRI), axial,
sequence 1

Sequence 2 coronal

T2-weighted, fat-saturated

Example

1.5 and 1.0 T: *HASTE sequence:*
TSE, FS, breathhold: — TR = 11.9
— TR = 3000–4000   — TE = 95
— TE = 100–140   — Flip angle 150°
(1.0 and) 0.5 T:
TSE, FS, respiratory triggering:
— TR = 1666 or 2500 (2–3 respirations)
— TE = 100
or

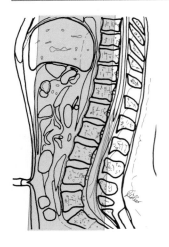

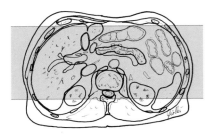

Small intestine (hydro-MRI),
coronal, sequence 3

— Slice thickness. 6 mm
— Slice gap: 20% of slice thickness ($\triangleq$ 1.2 mm or factor 1.2)
— FOV: large (at least 35 cm in order to avoid foldover), about 450 mm
— Saturation slab: no

Sequence 3 axial

T1-weighted

Example	
1.5 T:	*1.0 T:*
GRE (FLASH), breathhold:	*TSE (turbo factor) 3, breathhold:*
— TR = 120–140	— TR = 300
— TE = 4	— TE = 12
— Flip angle 60°	— If necessary, repeat 3–4 times until all of the small intestine has been imaged
1.0 T:	
— TR = 150–200	
— TE = 6	*0.5 T:*
— Flip angle 70°	*SE, respiratory compensation:*
or	— TR = 500–600
	— TE = 10–20
	— Flip angle 90°

otherwise as sequence 1

Sequence 4 coronal

T1-weighted

Example

1.5 T:	*1.0 T:*
GRE (FLASH), breathhold:	*TSE, breathhold:*
— TR = 120–140	— TR = 300
— TE = 4	— TE = 12
— Flip angle 60°	— If necessary, repeat 3–4 times until all of the small intestine has been imaged
1.0 T:	*0.5 T:*
— TR = 150–200	*SE, respiratory compensation:*
— TE = 6	— TR = 500–600
— Flip angle 70°	— TE = 10–20
or	— Flip angle 90°

---

otherwise as sequence 2

If needed, also:
— Injection of hyoscine butylbromide 20 mg
  and then
— I.v. bolus of Gd-DTPA 0.1 mmol/kg body weight
  followed by

Sequences 5–7 coronal

T1-weighted (as sequence 4; 20 seconds, 55 seconds, and 88 seconds after the injection starts)

Sequence 8 axial

T1-weighted (as sequence 3, but with fat saturation)

Sequence 9 coronal

T1-weighted (as sequence 4, but with fat saturation)

Modifications

MRI of the Small Intestine

— Performed after regular double contrast study of the small intestine

Patient Preparation
— Bowel evacuant (e.g. senna-based laxatives) in the afternoon and fluid intake (plenty to drink) in the evening on the day before the study
— Fasting on the day of the study

Materials
— Tube for small intestine enteroclysis (e.g., disposable Bilbao or Sellink tube)
— Suitable guide wire
— Topical anesthetic jelly or spray (e.g., xylocaine) for nasal or oral tube placement
— Two large-volume syringes
— Two containers for the contrast agent and the methylcellulose
— Adapter to link syringe and tube
  or
— Contrast pump, supply containers for the contrast agent and the methylcellulose with suitable tubing
— Tube for contrast pump
— Contrast and distention agent: 200 (up to 500) ml dilute contrast agent (specific weight 1.2–1.3, e.g., Micropaque fluid diluted with water, ratio 1:2)
— 1200 (up to 2000) ml methylcellulose (dissolve 10 g in 0.2 l water heated to about 60° and mix well, add 1800 ml cold water and remix)
— Instillation temperature: 18 °C (or body temperature)
— Add 100 ml of a Gd-containing oral contrast agent (e.g., Magnevist enteral, Schering, Berlin) to the methylcellulose

Technique
— Plain fluoroscopy
  is performed first
— After topical anesthesia of the nose and pharynx, the tube (kept rigid by the guide wire) is inserted through the nose with the patient standing
— The tube is further inserted; it may be necessary to lower the patient to the horizontal (right lateral decubitus first for passage through the pylorus; left lateral decubitus position for passage through the duodenum; the tip of the tube should be flexible)

— Standard placement of the distal tube is beyond the duodenojejunal junction (to avoid any reflux)
— The contrast agent is speedily instilled, initially under fluoroscopy (rate 80 ml/min, volume usually about 200 ml)
— MRI follows (sequences as described above, but after injection of hyoscine butylbromide 20 mg)

Pancreas

Patient Preparation
— Have the patient drink superparamagnetic (negative) contrast solution
— Have the patient go to the toilet before the study
— Explain the procedure to the patient
— Have the patient undress except for underwear
— Ask the patient to remove anything containing metal (hearing aids, hair-pins, body jewelry, etc.)
— Have an intravenous line placed

Positioning
— Supine
— Body array coil or body coil
— Cushion the legs
— If necessary, offer the patient ear protectors

Sequences
— Scout: axial and sagittal (three planes, if possible)

Sequence 1 coronal

T2-weighted

Example

1.5 and 1.0 T:	(1.0 and) 0.5 T:
TSE, breathhold:	TSE, respiratory triggering:
— TR = 3000–4000	— TR = 1900–2300
— TE = 90–140	— TE = 80–100
	— Flip angle 90°

— Slice thickness: 6–8 mm
— Slice gap: 20% of slice thickness ($\triangleq$ 1.2–1.6 mm or factor 1.2)
— FOV: 380–400 mm
— Saturation slab: axial superior to the slices for saturation of the vessels

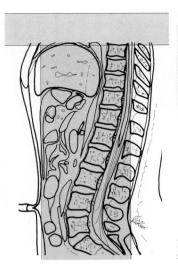
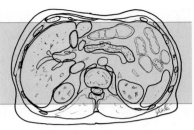

Pancreas, coronal,
sequence 1

Sequence 2 axial (plot on coronal slice across pancreas)

T2-weighted, fat-saturated

Example

1.5 and 1.0 T:	*(1.5 and) 0.5 T:*
TSE, FS, breathhold:	*TSE, respiratory triggering:*
— TR = 3000–4000	— TR = 1900–2300
— TE = 90–140	— TE = 80–100
— Flip angle 180°	— Flip angle 90°

— Slice thickness: 5–6 mm
— Slice gap: 20% of slice thickness ($\triangleq$ 1.0–1.2 mm or factor 1.2)
— FOV: 380–400 mm
— Saturation slab: axial (parallel) superior to the slices for saturation of the vessels and ventral (coronal) for saturation of the subcutaneous fat

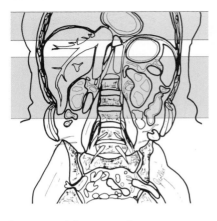 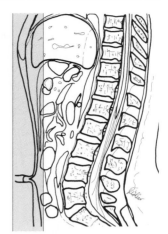

Pancreas, axial, sequence 2

Sequence 3 axial

T1-weighted, fat-saturated

Example

1.5 T:
GRE (FLASH), breathhold:
— TR = 120–140
— TE = 4
— Flip angle 60°
1.0 T:
GRE (FLASH), breathhold:
— TR = 120–140
— TE = 6–7 (in phase)
— Flip angle 60°
  or

1.0 and 0.5 T:
GRE (FLASH), respiratory compensation:
— TR = 500–600
— TE = 10–12
— Flip angle 90°

otherwise as sequence 2

Sequence 4 axial

T1-weighted, fat-saturated (as sequence 3, but after administration of Gd-DTPA)

and possibly

Sequence 5 coronal

T1-weighted, fat-saturated (after administration of contrast agent)

Example

1.5 and 1.0 T:
TSE, breathhold, GRE (FLASH):
— TR = 120–140
— TE = 4
— Flip angle 60°
or

FFE:
— TR = 15
— TE = 4
— Flip angle 25°
1.0 and 0.5 T:
Respiratory compensation:
— TR = 500–600
— TE = 10
— Flip angle 90°

— Slice thickness: 5–6 mm
— Slice gap: contiguous
— Saturation slab: axial (parallel) superior to the slices for saturation of the vessels

---

Tips & Tricks
— Hyoscine butylbromide 20 mg can be given intravenously to attenuate intestinal motility
— If there is a problem delineating the head of the pancreas from the duodenum, have the patient drink superparamagnetic contrast solution (e.g., Lumirem)
— Or have the patient drink a large glass of water immediately before the study
— Image the patient in the right lateral decubitus position

Modifications

Biliary Tree and Pancreatic Duct

Sequence 5 paracoronal (adjusted to the course of the pancreatic duct and the common bile duct = approx. 0–30° off the horizontal plane, plot on axial image)

T2-weighted, fat-saturated

Example	
1.5 and 1.0 T:	*0.5 T:*
HASTE:	*3-D IR-SE, respiratory triggering:*
— TR = 11.9	— TR = 1666 or 2500 respectively
— TE = 95	— TE = 700
— Flip angle 150°	— TI = 90

— Slice thickness = 4 mm with 50 % overlap = 2 mm
— Followed by MIP analysis
or

Single-slice technique: T2-weighted, fat-saturated, long TE, large turbo factor

Example	
1.5 and 1.0 T:	*(1.0 and) 0.5 T:*
(RARE sequence with large	*2-D TSE, FS (SPIR):*
turbo factor):	— TR = 8000
— TR = 2800	— TE = 1250
— TE = 1100	— Flip angle 90°
— Flip angle 150°	— Slice thickness = 70 mm
	— No MIP analysis required

— FOV: large (at least 35 cm in order to avoid foldover)

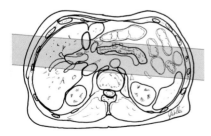

Biliary tree and pancreatic duct, paracoronal, sequence 5

Tips & Tricks
  — In sequence 5, run single-slice sequence as localizer first, because:
  • The sequence is very fast
  • The multislice sequence is then much more certain

Dynamic Contrast Series

E.g., when investigating for gastrinoma

Sequences

Sequences 1–3

as basic sequences (see above)

Sequence 4 axial

T1-weighted, breathhold, fat-saturated
(20 seconds after i. v. administration of Gd-DTPA) as basic sequence 3 (see above)

Sequence 5 axial

T1-weighted, breathhold, fat-saturated
(approx. 60 seconds after i. v. administration of Gd-DTPA) as basic sequence 3 (see above)

Sequence 6 axial

T1-weighted, breathhold, fat-saturated
(approx. 3 minutes after i. v. administration of Gd-DTPA) as basic sequence 3 (see above)

Secretin-Enhanced MR Pancreatography

— Slow (at least 1 minute) i. v. injection of secretin 1 U/kg body weight

Sequence 5

Single-slice technique: T2-weighted, fat-saturated, long TE, large turbo factor
(3 minutes after injection)

Example	
1.5 and 1.0 T:	or
— TR = 2800	*(1.0 and) 0.5 T:*
— TE = 1100	*2-D TSE, FS (SPIR):*
— Flip angle 150°	— TR = 8000
	— TE = 1250
	— Flip angle 90°
	— Slice thickness = 70 mm
	— FOV: large (at least 35 cm)

— No MIP analysis required

Sequence 6

If the duct has not been well delineated yet, repeat the scan 6 minutes after secretin injection

Kidney

Patient Preparation
— Have the patient go to the toilet before the study
— Explain the procedure to the patient
— Ask the patient to undress except for underwear
— Ask the patient to remove anything containing metal (hearing aids, hair-pins, body jewelry, etc.)
— Have an intravenous line placed

Positioning
— Supine
— Body array coil or body coil
— Cushion the legs
— If necessary, offer the patient ear protectors

Sequences
— Scout: axial, sagittal, and coronal

Sequence 1 coronal

T2-weighted

Example

1.5 and 1.0 T:
TSE, breathhold:
— TR = 3000–4000
— TE = 90–140
— Flip angle 180°
(1.0 and) 0.5 T:
TSE, respiratory triggering:
— TR = 1900–2300

— TE = 100
— Flip angle 90°
or
STIR:
— TR = 2200
— TE = 60
— TI = 100
— Flip angle 90°
or
HASTE, breathhold:
— TR = 11.9
— TE = 95
— Flip angle 150°

— Slice thickness: 4–6 mm
— Slice gap: 20% of slice thickness ($\triangleq$ 0.8–1.2 mm or factor 1.2)
— Phase encoding gradient: LR
— FOV: 380–400 mm
— Saturation slab: axial superior to the slices for saturation of the vessels

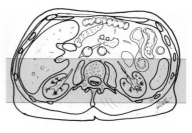

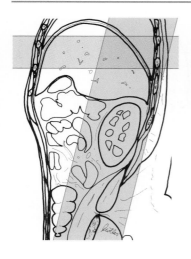

Kidney, coronal,
sequence 1

Sequence 2 axial

T2-weighted

Example

1.5 and 1.0 T:
TSE, breathhold:
— TR = 3000–4000
— TE = 90–140
— Flip angle 180°

(1.0 and) 0.5 T:
TSE, respiratory triggering:
— TR = 1900–2300
— TE = 100
— Flip angle 90°
— If spectral presaturation (SPIR) is used, TE may be reduced to 80 ms = stronger signal

---

— Slice thickness: 5–6 mm
— Slice gap: 0–20 % of slice thickness ($\triangleq$ 0–1.2 mm or factor 1.0–1.2)
— FOV: 380–400 mm (possibly rectangular FOV)
— Saturation slab: axial (parallel) superior to the slices for saturation of the vessels and ventral (coronal) for saturation of the subcutaneous fat

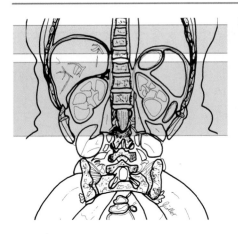

Kidney, axial, sequence 2

Sequence 3 axial

T1-weighted, otherwise as sequence 2 (possibly plus fat saturation)

Example

1.5 (1.0) T:
GRE (FFE), breathhold:
— TR = 120–140
— TE = 4 (1.0 T: 6–7)
— Flip angle 60°
(1.0 and) 0.5 T:
GRE (FFE), respiratory compensation:
— TR = 500–600
— TE = 10
— Flip angle 90°

or as SPIR:
— TR = 500–600
— TE = 15
— Flip angle 90°
or
TSE, breathhold:
— TR = 320
— TE = 14
— Matrix = 140 × 256
— Half-Fourier
— 9 slices

Sequence 4 axial

T1-weighted, otherwise as sequence 3 but after administration of contrast agent (Gd-DTPA 0.1 mmol/kg body weight)

Tips & Tricks
— If necessary, hyoscine butylbromide 20 mg can be given intravenously to attenuate intestinal motility
— If necessary, have the patient practice breathholding

Modifications

MR Urography

Patient Preparation
— Have the patient go to the toilet before the study
— Explain the procedure to the patient
— Have the patient undress except for underwear
— Ask the patient to remove anything containing metal (hearing aids, hair-pins, body jewelry, etc.)
— Have an intravenous line placed

Positioning
— Supine
— Body array coil or body coil
— Cushion the legs
— If necessary, offer the patient ear protectors

Preparation in the examination room
— Inject furosemide 0.1 mg/kg body weight i. v. (up to 5 mg if obstruction is suspected)
— 30–60 seconds after the furosemide injection administer the contrast agent (Gd-DTPA 0.1 mmol/kg body weight i. v.)

Sequences
— Scout: axial, sagittal, and coronal (three planes)

Sequence 1 paracoronal

(5–10 minutes after administration of the contrast agent)

T2-weighted, Half-Fourier (RARE), single-shot TSE with breathholding

Example	
— TR = 2900	*1.0 and 0.5 T:*
— TE = 200	— TR = 8000
— TF = 174	— TE = 1200
or	— TF = 255

— Slice thickness: 60–100 mm (single-slice technique in 8 seconds)
— FOV: large (e.g., 450 mm)
— Saturation slab: no

Sequence 2 paracoronal

T1-weighted (3-D spoiled GRE sequence, 3-D FLASH), fat-saturated

---

Example

1.5 T:
Breathhold:
— TR = 40
— TE = 7.6
— Flip angle 70°
or
T1-weighted angiography
sequence:
3-D GRE (FISP):
— TR = 6.8
— TE = 2.3

— Slab thickness = 60 mm
— Flip angle 45°
— No. of partitions = 28
— FOV: large (500 mm)
— Matrix = 512 (256)
1.0 and 0.5 T:
Respiratory compensation:
— TR = briefest (e.g., 72)
— TE = 7.6
— Flip angle 70°

— Slice thickness: 2 mm (50% overlap)
— FOV: large (e.g., 450 mm)
— Saturation slab: coronal, parallel to the slices

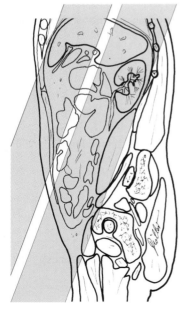

MR urography, paracoronal,
sequences 1 and 2

Adrenal Gland

Patient Preparation
— Have the patient go to the toilet before the study
— Explain the procedure to the patient
— Ask the patient to undress except for underwear
— Ask the patient to remove anything containing metal (hearing aids, hair-pins, body jewelry, etc.)
— Have an intravenous line placed

Positioning
— Supine
— Body array coil or body coil
— Cushion the legs
— If necessary, offer the patient ear protectors

Sequences
— Scout: axial, sagittal, and coronal

Sequence 1 coronal

T2-weighted

Example
1.5 and 1.0 T:
TSE, breathhold:
— TR = 3000–4500
— TE = 130–150
— Flip angle 180°
1.0 and 0.5 T:
TSE, respiratory triggering:
— TR = 1900

— TE = 100
— Flip angle 90°
  or
(1.5–0.5 T):
STIR:
— TR = 2200
— TE = 60
— TI = 100
— Flip angle 90°

— Slice thickness: 4–6 mm
— Slice gap: 0–20% of slice thickness ($\triangleq$ 0–1.2 mm or factor 1.0–1.2)
— Phase encoding gradient: FH (possibly with phase oversampling)
— FOV: 380–400 mm
— Saturation slab: axial superior to the slices for saturation of the vessels

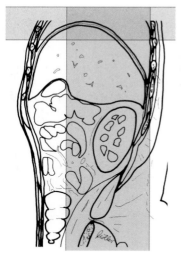

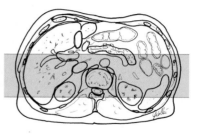

Adrenal gland, coronal,
sequence 1

Sequence 2 axial

T2-weighted

> **Example**
> *1.5 and 1.0 T:*
> *TSE, breathhold:*
> — TR = 3000–4500
> — TE = 130–150
> *1.0 and 0.5 T:*
> *TSE, respiratory triggering:*
> — TR = 1900–2300
> — TE = 100
> — Flip angle 90°

- Slice thickness: 5–6 mm
- Slice gap: 20% of slice thickness (≙ 1.0–1.2 mm or factor 1.2)
- Phase encoding gradient: AP
- FOV: 380–400 mm (possibly rectangular FOV)
- Saturation slab: axial (parallel) superior to the slices for saturation of the vessels and ventral (coronal) for saturation of the subcutaneous fat

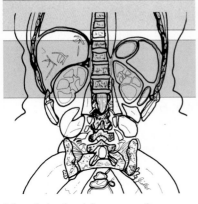
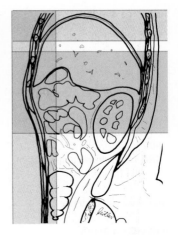

Adrenal gland, axial, sequence 2

Sequence 3 axial

GRE in phase

Example	
1.5 (1.0) T:	— TE = 6.9
GRE, breathhold:	— Flip angle 25°
— TR = 70–170	*0.5 T:*
— TE = 4–5 (1.0 T: 6–7)	*GRE, respiratory compensation:*
— Flip angle 60–90°	— TR = 15
1.0 T:	— TE = 3.45
GRE, respiratory compensation:	— Flip angle 25°
— TR = 15	

otherwise as sequence 2.

Sequence 4 axial

GRE out of phase

Example
1.5 (1.0) T: — TE = 3.45
GRE, breathhold: — Flip angle 25°
— TR = 70–170   *0.5 T:*
— TE = 2–3/6–7 (1.0 T: 3.5/10)   *GRE, breathhold:*
— Flip angle 60–90°   — TR = 15
1.0 T: — TE = 6.9
GRE, respiratory compensation: — Flip angle 25°
— TR = 15

---

otherwise as sequence 2

Sequence 5 axial

T1-weighted, noncontrast

Example
1.5 T: — TE = 10
GRE (FLASH), breathhold: — Flip angle 90°
— TR = 30–40   or
— TE = 16   *SPIR:*
— Flip angle 70°   — TR = 500–600
1.0 and 0.5 T: — TE = 15
GRE (FLASH), respiratory   — Flip angle 90°
compensation:
— TR = 500–600

---

otherwise as sequence 2

Tips & Tricks
— Hyoscine butylbromide may be injected intravenously to attenuate in-
  testinal motility
— If necessary, have the patient practice breathholding

Modifications

Dynamic Series

Sequences

Sequences 1–4
as above

Sequence 5 axial

T1-weighted, noncontrast

Example
1.5 and 1.0 T: — TE = 4.8
GRE (FLASH), breathhold: — Flip angle 80°
— TR = 70–170   or
— TE = 4–5 (1.0 T: 6–7)   *T1 turbo-field:*
— Flip angle 70°   — TR = 13
1.0 and 0.5 T: — TE = 4.5–5
FFE, respiratory compensation: — Flip angle 25°
— TR = 170

---

otherwise as basic sequence 2

Sequences 6–11 axial

T1-weighted, dynamic = 30 seconds, 1 minute, 2 minutes, 5 minutes, and 10 minutes after intravenous administration of contrast agent

---

Example
Gd-DTPA 0.1 mmol/kg body
weight: — TE = 4.8
1.5 and 1.0 T: — Flip angle 80°
GRE (FLASH), breathhold: or
— TR = 70–170   *T1 turbo-field:*
— TE = 4–5 (1.0 T: 6–7)   — TR = 13
— Flip angle 70°   — TE = 4.5–5
1.0 and 0.5 T: — Flip angle 25°
FFE, respiratory compensation:
— TR = 170

---

otherwise as basic sequence 2

Pelvis

Patient Preparation
— *Do not* have the patient go to the toilet before the study (the bladder must be full)
— Explain the procedure to the patient
— Offer the patient ear protectors or ear plugs
— Ask the patient to undress above the waist except for underwear
— Ask the patient to remove anything containing metal (hearing aids, hairpins, body jewelry, etc.)
— Depending on the purpose of the investigation, have the patient drink negative contrast solution (e.g., Lumirem)
— If necessary, have an intravenous line placed

Positioning

— Supine
— Body array coil (wraparound) or body coil
— Cushion the legs
— Arms folded on the chest

Sequences
— Scout: sagittal and coronal (three planes, if possible)

Sequence 1 axial

T2-weighted, possibly fat-saturated

Example
TSE, FS:
— TR = 2000–4500
— TE = 100–130
— TF = 18

— Slice thickness: 6 mm
— Slice gap: 20% of slice thickness ($\triangleq$ 1.2 mm or factor 1.2)
— Phase encoding gradient: LR
— FOV: ≤ 400 mm
— Matrix: possibly 512 (256)
— Saturation slab:
  - Axial (parallel) superior to the slices for saturation of the vessels
  - Ventral (coronal, orthogonal to the slices) for saturation of the fatty tissue of the abdominal wall

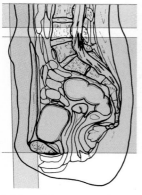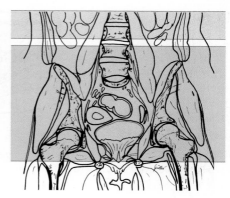

Pelvis, axial, sequence 1

Sequence 2 axial

T1-weighted

> **Example**
> *TSE:*   — Flip angle 90°, possibly 150°
> — TR = 500–700   — TF = 4
> — TE = 12–25

— Slice thickness: 8 mm
— Slice gap: 30% of slice thickness (≙ 2.4 mm or factor 1.3)
— Matrix: perhaps 512 (256)
— Saturation slab:
  - Axial superior to the slices for saturation of the vessels
  - Ventral (coronal, orthogonal to the slices) for saturation of the fatty tissue of the abdominal wall

Sequence 3 coronal

T2-weighted

> **Example**
> *TSE:*
> — TR = 2500–4500
> — TE = 100–130
> — TF = 16

— Slice thickness: 5–6 mm
— Slice gap: 30% of slice thickness (≙ 1.5–1.8 mm or factor 1.3)

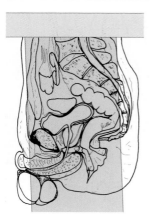
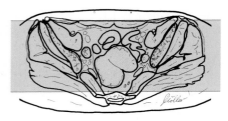

Pelvis, coronal,
sequence 3

— Phase encoding gradient: HF (or LR, particularly in the case of respiratory motion artifacts due to uncontrasted intestinal fluid
— Saturation slab: axial superior to the slices for saturation of the vessels

  and possibly

Sequence 4 axial

T1-weighted, as sequence 2 but after administration of contrast agent (Gd-DTPA)

Tips & Tricks
— Hyoscine butylbromide may be given intravenously to attenuate intestinal motility
— If necessary, secure strap across the abdomen to limit respiratory motion
— Ask the patient to breathe "only with your chest"

Modifications

Uterus, Vagina, Bladder

Sequences

Sequence 1 axial

T2-weighted (as basic sequence 1 above)

Sequence 2 axial

T1-weighted (as basic sequence 2 above)

Sequence 3 coronal
(allow for possible oblique position of the pelvis)

TIRM or STIR

Example

1.5 and 1.0 T:
— TR = 6500
— TE = 30–60
— TI = 140
— Flip angle 90°

(1.0 and) 0.5 T:
— TR = 1800
— TE = 60
— TI = 100
— Flip angle 90°

---

or

T2-weighted, fat-saturated

Example
TSE, FS:
— TR = 2500–3500
— TE = 100–130

— Slice thickness: 4 mm
— Slice gap: 0–20% of slice thickness ($\triangleq$ 0–0.8 mm or factor 1.0–1.2)
— Saturation slab: axial superior to the slices for saturation of the vessels

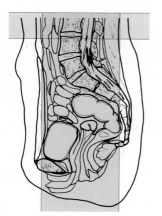
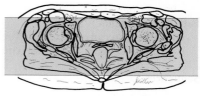

Uterus, vagina, bladder, coronal,
sequence 3

Sequence 4 sagittal

T2-weighted

> **Example**
> *TSE:*
> — TR = 2500–3500
> — TE = 100–130

- Slice thickness: 6 mm
- Slice gap: 10% of slice thickness (≙ 0 mm or factor 1.0)
- Matrix: 512 (256)
- Saturation slab: no

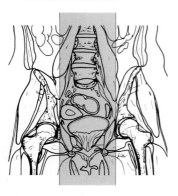
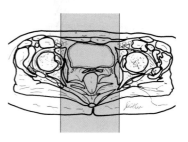

Uterus, vagina, bladder, sagittal, sequence 4

Prostate

Patient Preparation
- Possibly endorectal or circular surface coil (in thin patients: place on ventral surface of pelvis and secure with strap, use small FOV)

Sequences

Sequence 1 axial

superior to the pelvic floor (plot on sagittal scout)

T2-weighted

> **Example**
> *TSE:*   — Matrix = 512
> — TR = 2500–4500
> — TE = 100–130

- Slice thickness: 3–4 mm
- Slice gap: 20 % of slice thickness ($\triangleq$ 0.8 mm or factor 1.2)
- FOV: 250–300 mm
- Two saturation slabs:
  - Axial (parallel) superior to the slices for saturation of the vessels
  - Ventral (coronal, orthogonal to the slices) for saturation of the fatty tissue of the abdominal wall

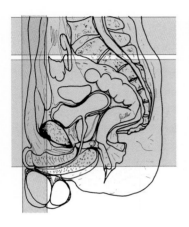
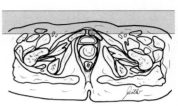

Prostate, axial superior to the pelvic floor, sequence 1

or (if just the prostate is being investigated and there already are studies of the pelvis)

Sequence 1 axial across the prostate (plot on sagittal scout)

T2-weighted

> **Example**
> *TSE:* — TE = 100–130
> — TR = 2500–4500

- Slice thickness: 3 mm
- Slice gap: 0–20 % of slice thickness ($\triangleq$ 0–0.6 mm or factor 1.0–1.2)
- FOV: 150–200 mm
- NSA: 6–8
- Phase encoding gradient: AP (or LR, but then with phase oversampling)
- Matrix: 512
- Two saturation slabs:
  - Axial (parallel) superior to the slices for saturation of the vessels
  - Ventral (coronal, orthogonal to the slices) for saturation of the fatty tissue of the abdominal wall

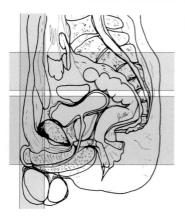

Prostate, axial across the prostate, sequence 1

Sequence 2 coronal

T2-weighted

Example
TSE:
— TR = 2500–4500
— TE = 100–130

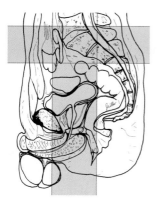 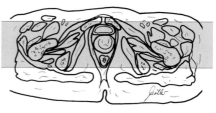

Prostate, coronal,
sequence 2

— Slice thickness: 3 mm
— Slice gap: 0–20% of slice thickness ($\triangleq$ 0–0.6 mm or factor 1.0–1.2)
— FOV: small (e.g., 200–250 mm with phase oversampling)
— NSA: 6–8
— Matrix: 512 (256)
— Saturation slab: axial superior to the slices for saturation of the vessels

Sequence 3 axial

T1-weighted

> **Example**
> — TR = 500–700
> — TE = 12–20

— Slice thickness: 3 mm
— Slice gap: 0–20% of slice thickness ($\triangleq$ 0–0.6 mm or factor 1.0–1.2)
— FOV: 200–250 mm
— Matrix: 256 or 512, but then with NSA 4–6 for improved signal-to-noise ratio
— Saturation slab:
  ◦ Axial superior to the slices for saturation of the vessels
  ◦ Ventral (coronal, orthogonal to the slices) for saturation of the fatty tissue of the abdominal wall

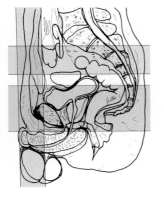

Prostate, axial, sequence 3

Sequence 4 axial

T1-weighted, as sequence 2 but after administration of contrast agent (Gd-DTPA)

and possibly

Sequence 5 coronal or sagittal across the prostate

T1-weighted

> **Example**
> — TR = 500–700   — Flip angle 90°, possibly 150°
> — TE = 12–25

— Slice thickness 3 mm
— Slice gap: 0–20% of slice thickness (≙ 0–0.6 mm or factor 1.0–1.2)
— Matrix: 512
— Saturation slab: axial superior to the slices for saturation of the vessels

Pelvic Outlet Measurements (Sizing the Birth Canal)

Sequences

Sequence 1 sagittal

T2-weighted

> **Example**
> *TSE:*
> — TR = 1800–3000
> — TE = 100–130

— Slice thickness: 8 mm
— Slice gap: 20% of slice thickness (≙ 1.6 mm or factor 1.2)
— Only a few slices are needed

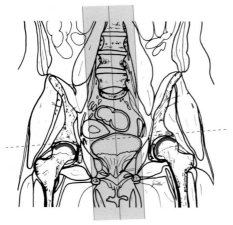

Pelvic outlet measurements (sizing the birth canal), sagittal, sequence 1

Sequence 2 paracoronal

T2-weighted along the true conjugate diameter (plot on mediosagittal slice = line between promontory and posterior aspect of the symphysis pubis), otherwise as sequence 1 (only a few slices are needed)

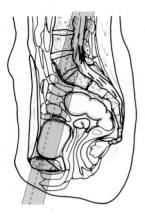

Pelvic outlet measurements (sizing the birth canal), paracoronal, sequence 2

Sequence 3 axial

T2-weighted (from the posterior aspect of the symphysis pubis to the coccygeal bone; *note:* image the pelvic outlet as well), otherwise as sequence 1 (only a few slices are needed)

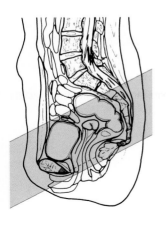

Pelvic outlet measurements (sizing the birth canal), axial, sequence 3

Testes

Patient Preparation
— Have the patient go to the toilet before the study
— Explain the procedure to the patient
— Offer the patient ear protectors or ear plugs
— Ask the patient to undress except for underwear
— Ask the patient to remove anything containing metal (hearing aids, hairpins, body jewelry, etc.)
— Have an intravenous line placed

Positioning

— Supine
— Body array coil (wraparound coil, surface coil, e.g., circular surface coil)
— Cushion the legs

Sequences
— Scout: coronal, sagittal, and axial

Sequence 1 coronal

T2-weighted

Example
TSE:
— TR = 2000–4000
— TE = 100–150

— Slice thickness: 4 mm
— Slice gap: 0–20% of slice thickness ($\triangleq$ 0–0.8 mm or factor 1.0–1.2)
— FOV: small (e.g., 200 mm)
— Matrix: 512 (but then with NSA 3–4)
— Phase oversampling
— Saturation slab: axial superior to the slices for saturation of the vessels

Sequence 2 coronal

T1-weighted

Example
— TR = 500–600
— TE = 12–25

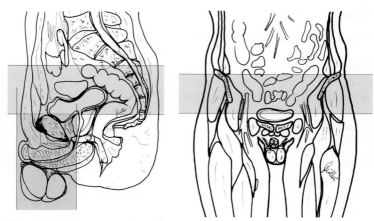

Testes, coronal, sequences 1 and 2

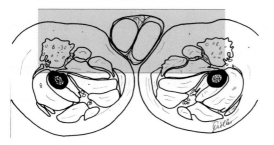

Testes, axial, sequence 4

— Slice thickness: 4 mm
— Slice gap: 0–20% of slice thickness (≙ 0–0.8 mm or factor 1.0–1.2)
— FOV: small (e.g., 200 mm)
— Phase oversampling
— Saturation slab: axial superior to the slices for saturation of the vessels

Sequence 3 coronal

As sequence 2 but after administration of contrast agent (Gd-DTPA)

Sequence 4 axial

T1-weighted
after administration of contrast agent

Example
— TR = 500–700
— TE = 10–20

— Slice thickness: 4 mm
— Slice gap: 20% of slice thickness ($\triangleq$ 0.8 mm or factor 1.2)
— FOV: small (e.g., 200 mm)
— Saturation slab: axial superior to the slices for saturation of the vessels

Tips & Tricks
— Positioning aid: leave tight-fitting underpants in place (immobilizes the testes)
— If necessary, cushion the testes
— If a surface coil is used, perhaps place a thin foam pad between testes and coil to prevent too strong a signal in the vicinity of the coil

Magnetic Resonance Imaging:
Bones, Joints

Temporomandibular Joint

Patient Preparation
— Thirty minutes before the study administer Gd-DTPA 0.2 mmol/kg body weight (about 10–20 ml) intravenously (indirect arthrography)
— Have the patient chew gum intensely for at least 20 minutes
— Have the patient go to the toilet before the study
— Ask the patient to remove anything containing metal (hearing aids, hairpins, body jewelry, necklace, etc.)
— Explain the procedure to the patient:
  - Check to see how far the patient can open his/her mouth
  - Fashion bite block (the mouth has to stay in maximum open position for several minutes), if not already done
  - Practice fitting in the bite block with the patient

Positioning
— Supine
— Temporomandibular joint (TMJ) double coil (or head coil, or eye-ear coil or surface coil: e.g., flexible coil: position the head of the patient on the flexible coil, flip up the coil on the left and right side of the head and secure with straps)

Sequences
— Scout 1: axial and coronal (three planes, if possible)
— Scout 2: sagittal and coronal (especially of the TMJs set up on the first scout)

Sequence 1 (para-) coronal across each mandibular condyle (adjusted to the oblique position of the condyle = approx. 20° off the horizontal plane), mouth closed

T1-weighted

Example	
SE:	— TE = 7 (1.5 T) or 10 (1.0 T)
— TR = 400–500	— Flip angle 30°
— TE = 10–15	or
— Flip angle 90°, possibly 60°	*0.5 T:*
or	*3-D FFE:*
1.5 and 1.0 T:	— TR = 30
GRE:	— TE = 13
— TR = 300–400	— Flip angle 30°

— Slice thickness: 2 mm

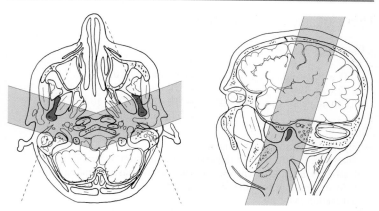

Temporomandibular joint, (para-) coronal across each mandibular condyle, sequence 1

— Slice gap: 0–20% of slice thickness ($\triangleq$ 0–0.4 mm or factor 1.0–1.2)
— Phase encoding gradient: LR (possibly with phase oversampling)
— FOV: as small as possible (e.g., 120 mm)
— Saturation slab: no

Sequence 2 (para-) sagittal across each mandibular condyle (allowing for the oblique position of the mandibular ramus = approx. 70° and 110° respectively off the horizontal plane), mouth closed

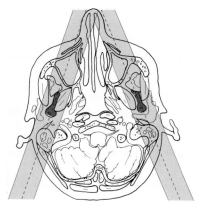

Temporomandibular joint, (para-) sagittal across each mandibular condyle, sequence 2

T1-weighted

Example

SE:	or
— TR = 400–500	*GRE: (1.5 and 1.0 T):*
— TE = 10–15	— TR = 300–400
— Flip angle 90°, possibly 60°	— TE = 7 (1.5 T) or 10 (1.0 T)
	— Flip angle 30°

— Slice thickness: 2 mm
— Slice gap: 0–20% of slice thickness ($\triangleq$ 0–0.4 mm or factor 1.0–1.2)
— Phase encoding gradient: AP (possibly with phase oversampling)
— FOV: as small as possible (e.g., 120 mm)
— Saturation slab: no
Ask the patient to open his/her mouth as far as possible and secure this position with the bite block while trying to keep the head in position

Sequence 3 (para-) sagittal, as sequence 2 but with the mouth open and secured by bite block

Sequence 4 (para-) sagittal, as sequence 2 (mouth closed) but:

T2-weighted

Example

TSE:
— TR = 2000–3500
— TE = 100–120

— Slice thickness: 3 mm
— Slice gap: 0–20% of slice thickness ($\triangleq$ 0–0.6 mm or factor 1.0–1.2)

Tips & Tricks
— If at all possible, briefly practice fitting in the bite block with the patient in the coil; the patient should not move his/her head
— If possible, for parasagittal imaging the tilt should be such that the slices do not pass through the sigmoid sinus (in order to avoid flow artifacts)
— Otherwise a (coronal) saturation slab through the sigmoid sinus may become necessary

Shoulder

Patient Preparation
— Have the patient to go to the toilet
— Explain the procedure to the patient
— Offer the patient ear protectors or ear plugs
— Ask the patient to undress except for underwear
— Ask the patient to remove anything containing metal (hearing aids, hair-pins, body jewelry, necklace, etc.)

Positioning
— Supine
— Shoulder coil (oval surface coil, flexible coil)
— Arm in neutral rotation or supination
— Cushion the legs

Sequences
— Scout: axial and coronal

Sequence 1 axial

T2-weighted, fat-saturated

Example

TSE, FS:
— TR = 2000–4500
— TE = 90–130
  or

GRE or, to delineate the glenoid labrum, FFE:
— TR = 600–700
— TE = 11
— Flip angle 60°

— Slice thickness: 3 mm (2-D), approx. 1 mm for GRE
— Slice gap: 20% of slice thickness ($\triangleq$ 0.6 mm or factor 1.2)
— FOV: 200–270 mm
— Saturation slab: no

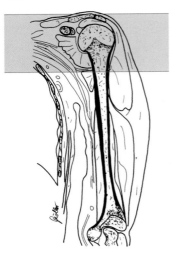

Shoulder, axial,
sequence 1

Sequence 2 paracoronal (parallel to the supraspinatus muscle on the axial slice)

T2-weighted, fat-saturated

Example	
TSE, FS:	*STIR:*
— TR = 2000–3500	— TR = 1800–2200
— TE = 100–120	— TE = 60
or	— TI = 100–130
	— Flip angle 90° each

— Slice thickness: 3 mm
— Slice gap: 20% of slice thickness ($\triangleq$ 0.6 mm or factor 1.2)
— FOV: approx. 260–290 mm
— Matrix: 512 (256)
— Saturation slab: parasagittal, oblique to the slice superior to the lung

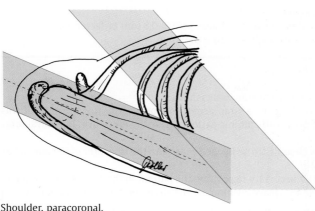

Shoulder, paracoronal,
sequence 2

Sequence 3 paracoronal

T1-weighted, otherwise as sequence 2

> **Example**
> — TR = 450–600
> — TE = 12–25

Sequence 4 parasagittal (orthogonal to sequence 2 or parallel to the glenoid cavity)

T1-weighted

> **Example**
> — TR = 500–600
> — TE = 10–20

or

T2-weighted

> **Example**
> — TR = 2000–4500
> — TE = 90–130

— Slice thickness: 3–4 mm
— Slice gap: 20 % of slice thickness ($\triangleq$ 0.6–0.8 mm or factor 1.2)
— Saturation slab: sagittal across the lungs

Tips & Tricks

— Positioning:
  Secure coil at the side with sandbags
  Place sandbags or a strap across the lower arm in supination (if this should prove difficult it is easier to have the lower arm in neutral rotation)
— Get the shoulder to be imaged as far into the isocenter of the magnet as possible
— It may be necessary to position the patient in the magnet at an oblique angle of 45° (place cushions at the shoulder, buttocks, and knees)

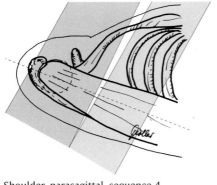
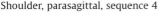
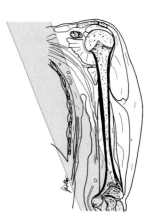

Shoulder, parasagittal, sequence 4

Modifications

Indirect Arthrography of the Shoulder
(e.g., for diagnostic workup of the glenoid labrum)

Patient Preparation
— Thirty minutes before the study administer Gd-DTPA 0.2 mmol/kg body weight (about 10–20 ml) intravenously
— Have the patient move the shoulder

Sequences

Sequence 1 axial (slice position as for basic sequence 1)

T1-weighted, fat-saturated

Example	
TSE, FS:	*GRE:*
— TR = 600–800	— TR = 400–500
— TE = 12–25	— TE = minimum
or	— Flip angle 80–90°

— Slice thickness: 3 mm
— Slice gap: 20% of slice thickness ($\triangleq$ 0.6 mm or factor 1.2)
— Matrix: 512
— FOV: 200–220 mm
— Saturation slab: no

Sequence 2 paracoronal

T2-weighted (as sequence 2)

Sequence 3 paracoronal

T1-weighted, fat-saturated (otherwise as sequence 3)

Sequence 4 parasagittal

T1-weighted, fat-saturated (otherwise as sequence 4)

Upper Arm

Patient Preparation
— Have the patient go to the toilet before the study
— Explain the procedure to the patient
— Offer the patient ear protectors or ear plugs
— Ask the patient to undress except for underwear
— Ask the patient to remove anything containing metal (hearing aids, hair-pins, body jewelry, etc.)

Positioning
— Supine
— Body coil (wraparound coil, body array coil; if needed, wrap large flexible coil spirally around the upper arm, with the upper end positioned outside the shoulder and the lower end at the elbow. Advantage: this minimizes foldover)
— Arm at the side (position as far into the isocenter as possible)
— Raise and cushion the elbow

Sequences
— Scout: coronal and sagittal (three planes, if possible)

Sequence 1 coronal
TIRM or STIR

Example	
1.5 and 1.0 T:	*(1.5 and) 0.5 T:*
— TR = 6500	— TR = 1600–2100
— TE = 30–60	— TE = 60
— TI = 140	— TI = 100–140
— Flip angle 180°	— Flip angle 90°

or

T2-weighted, fat-saturated

Example
TSE, FS:
— TR = 2000–3500
— TE = 90–120

— Slice thickness: 4–5 mm
— Slice gap: 20% of slice thickness (≙ 0.8–1.0 mm or factor 1.2)
— Matrix: 512
— FOV: ≤ 400 mm
— Saturation slab: sagittal across the lungs and vessels

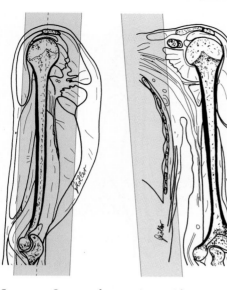

Upper arm, coronal,
sequence 1

Sequence 2 coronal, as sequence 1 but:

T1-weighted

> **Example**
> — TR = 500–600
> — TE = 10–25

Sequence 3 axial (the position of the slices depends on the pathologic findings or the purpose of the investigation)

T2-weighted

> **Example**
> *TSE:*
> — TR = 2000–4000
> — TE = 90–130

— Slice thickness: 5–6 mm
— Slice gap: 20–50% of slice thickness ($\triangleq$ 1.0–3 mm or factor 1.2–1.5)
— Phase encoding gradient: AP (for body array coil: HF with phase oversampling)
— FOV: ≤ 200 mm
— Saturation slab: axial (parallel) superior to the slices for saturation of the vessels

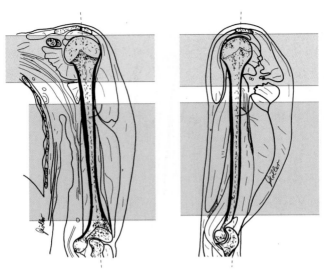

Upper arm, axial, sequence 3

Sequence 4 sagittal

T1-weighted

> **Example**
> — TR = 500–600
> — TE = 10–25

— Slice thickness: 5–6 mm
— Slice gap: 20% of slice thickness ($\triangleq$ 1.0–1.2 mm or factor 1.2)
— FOV: ≤ 400 mm
— Saturation slab: no

and possibly

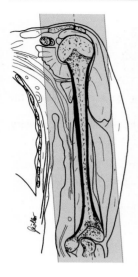 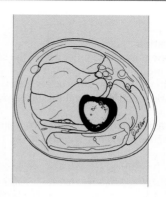

Upper arm, sagittal, sequence 4

Sequence 5 sagittal as sequence 4 but after administration of intravenous contrast agent (Gd-DTPA 0.2 mmol/kg body weight)

Sequence 6 axial (across the region in question)

T1-weighted

Example
— TR = 500–600
— TE = 10–25

— Slice thickness. 5–6 mm
— Slice gap: 20 % of slice thickness ($\triangleq$ 1.0–1.2 mm or factor 1.2)
— FOV: $\leq$ 200 mm
— Saturation slab: axial (parallel) superior to the slices for saturation of the vessels

Tips & Tricks
— Position the patient obliquely
   Advantage: the arm to be imaged is in the isocenter of the magnet
— The position is more stable if the patient can lean back against the inside of the tunnel

Elbow

Patient Preparation
— Have the patient go to the toilet before the study
— Explain the procedure to the patient
— Offer the patient ear protectors or ear plugs
— Have the patient undress except for underwear (perhaps only above the waist)
— Ask the patient to remove anything containing metal (watch, jewelry, hearing aids, hairpins, body jewelry, etc.)

Positioning
— Prone: arms straight above the head, palms against the table, secure
— Or supine: arms straight alongside the body
— Or slight lateral decubitus: arm immobilized by the body
— Surface or wraparound coil

Sequences
— Scout: axial and sagittal (three planes, if possible)

Sequence 1 coronal (set up on axial and sagittal slice)

TIRM or STIR

Example	
1.5 and 1.0 T:	*(1.0 and) 0.5 T:*
— TR = 5000–6500	— TR = 1500–2200
— TE = 30–60	— TE = 30–60
— TI = 140	— TI = 100–120
— Flip angle 180°	— Flip angle 90°

or

T2-weighted, fat-saturated

Example
TSE, FS:
— TR = 2000–3500
— TE = 70–100

— Slice thickness: 3–4 mm
— Slice gap: 0–20% of slice thickness (≙ 0–0.8 mm or factor 1.0–1.2)
— FOV: 120–150 mm
— Matrix: 512, if possible
— Saturation slab: axial proximal to the slices (through the distal upper arm)

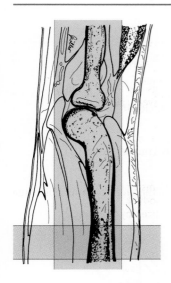
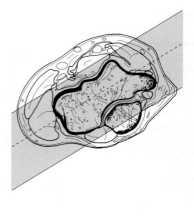

Elbow, coronal,
sequence 1

Sequence 2 coronal (as sequence 1)

T1-weighted

> **Example**
> — TR = 500–700
> — TE = 12–25

— Slice thickness: 3–4 mm
— Slice gap: 10–20 % of slice thickness ($\triangleq$ 0.3–0.8 mm or factor 1.1–1.2)
— FOV: 120–150 mm
— Matrix: 512, if possible
— Saturation slab: axial proximal to the slices (through the distal upper arm)

Sequence 3 axial

T2-weighted

> **Example**
> *TSE:*
> — TR = 2000–4000
> — TE = 100–130

or

T1-weighted

> **Example**
> — TR = 500–700
> — TE = 10–20
>
> *SPIR:*
> — TR = 2400
> — TE = 19
> — Flip angle 90°

— Slice thickness: 3–4 mm
— Slice gap: 20% of slice thickness (≙ 0.6–0.8 mm or factor 1.2)
— FOV: 120–150 mm
— Matrix: 512, if possible
— Saturation slab: axial (parallel) proximal to the slices for saturation of the vessels

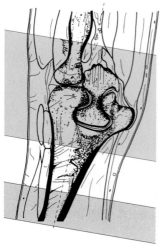 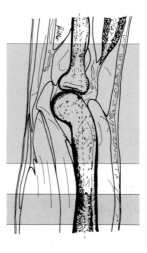

Elbow, axial, sequence 3

Sequence 4 sagittal

T2-weighted, 3-D GRE:

Example

DESS:	*FFE, fat-saturated:*
— TR = 25	— TR = 30–111
— TE = 9	— TE = 20–27
— Flip angle 35°	— Flip angle 15–25°

— Slab thickness: 60 mm (effective thickness approx. 0.9 mm)
— No. of partitions: 64
— Matrix: 512
— Saturation slab: axial proximal (orthogonal to the slices, no saturation for DESS)

Tips & Tricks
— If necessary, immobilize the forearm with a sandbag
— Try to position the elbow to be imaged in the isocenter of the magnet

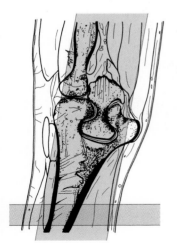 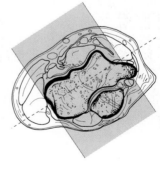

Elbow, sagittal,
sequence 4

Modifications

Indirect Arthrography of the Elbow (e.g., when looking for a loose body)

Patient Preparation
— Thirty minutes before the study, administer Gd-DTPA 0.2 mmol/kg body weight (about 10–20 ml) i. v.
— Have the patient move the arm

Sequences

Sequence 1 coronal

TIRM or STIR (as sequence 1)

Sequence 2 coronal

T1-weighted, fat-saturated (otherwise as sequence 2)

Sequence 3 axial

T1-weighted, fat-saturated (otherwise as sequence 3)
Sequence 4 sagittal

GRE (as sequence 4)

Forearm

Patient Preparation
— Have the patient go to the toilet before the study
— Explain the procedure to the patient
— Offer the patient ear protectors or ear plugs
— Ask the patient to undress except for underwear
— Ask the patient to remove anything containing metal (hearing aids, hair-pins, body jewelry, etc.)

Positioning
— Prone: arms extended above the head (wraparound coil)
— Supine: arm extended alongside the body
— Body coil (body array coil, wraparound coil: e.g., wrap large flexible coil around the forearm in spiral fashion)

Sequences
— Scout: axial and sagittal (three planes, if possible)

Sequence 1 coronal
TIRM or STIR

Example	
1.5 and 1.0 T:	*(1.0 and) 0.5 T:*
— TR = 5000–6500	— TR = 1800–2200
— TE = 30–60	— TE = 40–60
— TI = 140	— TI = 100–130
— Flip angle 180°	— Flip angle 90°

or

T2-weighted, fat-saturated

Example
TS, FS:
— TR = 2000–3500
— TE = 90–100

— Slice thickness: 4 mm
— Slice gap: 0–20% of slice thickness ($\triangleq$ 0–0.8 mm or factor 1.0–1.2)
— Phase encoding gradient: LR (HF for body array coil; possibly with phase oversampling)
— FOV: ≤ 400 mm

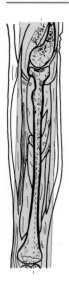

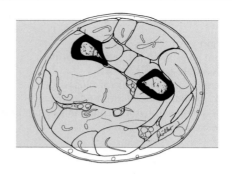

Forearm, coronal,
sequence 1

— Matrix: 512, if possible
— Saturation slab: axial superior to the slices for saturation of the vessels

Sequence 2 coronal

T1-weighted

> **Example**
> — TR = 500–600
> — TE = 10–20

— Slice thickness: 4 mm
— Slice gap: 20 % of slice thickness ($\triangleq$ 0.8 mm or factor 1.2)
— Matrix: 512, if possible
— FOV: ≤ 400 mm
— Saturation slab: axial superior to the slices for saturation of the vessels

Sequence 3 sagittal

T2-weighted

> **Example**
> *TSE:*
> — TR = 2000–4000
> — TE = 90–130

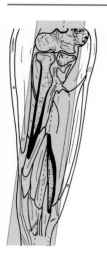 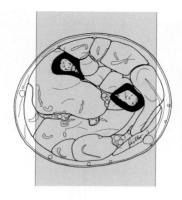

Forearm, sagittal,
sequence 3

— Slice thickness: 6–8 mm
— Slice gap: 20% of slice thickness (≙ 1.2–1.6 mm or factor 1.2)
— Saturation slab: axial superior to the slices for saturation of the vessels

Sequence 4 axial

T1-weighted

> **Example**
> — TR = 500–600
> — TE = 10–15

— Slice thickness: 6–8 mm
— Slice gap: 20–50% of slice thickness (≙ 1.2–4 mm or factor 1.2–1.5)
— FOV: ≤ 200 mm
— Saturation slab: axial (parallel) superior to the slices for saturation of the vessels

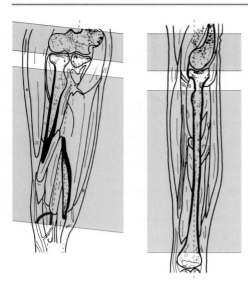

Forearm, axial, sequence 4

Sequence 5 axial as sequence 4 but after administration of intravenous contrast agent (Gd-DTPA 0.2 mmol/kg body weight)

Tips & Tricks
— If necessary, immobilize forearm with sandbag
— Study can also be performed with the patient prone, arm above the head and bent 90° at the elbow

Wrist

Patient Preparation
— Have the patient go to the toilet before the study
— Explain the procedure to the patient
— Offer the patient ear protectors or ear plugs
— Have the patient undress except for underwear (perhaps only above the waist)
— Ask the patient to remove anything containing metal (watch, jewelry, hearing aid, hairpins, body jewelry, etc.)

Positioning

— Prone: arm extended above the head, palm flat on the table, secure, surface coil
— Or supine: arm extended alongside the body

Sequences
— Scout: axial or sagittal

Sequence 1 coronal (set up on sagittal slice, adjust axis on axial slice)

TIRM or STIR

Example

1.5 and 1.0 T:	*(1.0 and) 0.5 T:*
— TR = 5000–6500	— TR = 1500–2200
— TE = 30–60	— TE = 30–60
— TI = 140	— TI = 100
— Flip angle 180°	— Flip angle 90°

or

T2-weighted, fat-saturated

Example
TSE, FS:
— TR = 2000–3500
— TE = 80–100

— Slice thickness: 3–4 mm
— Slice gap: 20% of slice thickness ($\triangleq$ 0.6–0.8 mm or factor 1.2)
— FOV: 120–150 mm
— Matrix: 512, if possible
— Saturation slab: axial proximal to the slices (across distal forearm)

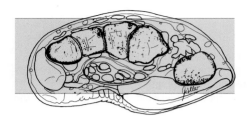

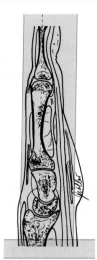

Wrist, coronal,
sequence 1

Sequence 2 coronal (as sequence 1)

T1-weighted

> **Example**
> *SE:*   *GRE:*
> — TR = 500–700   — TR = 400–600
> — TE = 10–20   — TE = minimum (≤ 11)
> or   — Flip angle 80–90°

— Slice thickness: 3–4 mm
— Slice gap: 0–10% of slice thickness ($\triangleq$ 0–0.4 mm or factor 1.0–1.1)
— FOV: 120–150 mm
— Matrix: 512, if possible
— Saturation slab: axial proximal to the slices (across the distal forearm)

Sequence 3 axial

T2-weighted

> **Example**
> *TSE:*
> — TR = 2000–4000
> — TE = 90–130

or

T1-weighted

> **Example**
> — TR = 500–700   *SPIR:*
> — TE = 10–20   — TR = 2400
> or   — TE = 19
>   — Flip angle 90°

— Slice thickness: 3–4 mm
— Slice gap: 20% of slice thickness ($\triangleq$ 0.6–0.8 mm or factor 1.2)
— FOV: 120–150 mm
— Matrix: 512, if possible
— Saturation slab: axial (parallel) proximal to the slices for saturation of the vessels

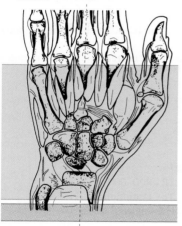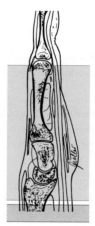

Wrist, axial, sequence 3

Sequence 4 coronal

T2-weighted, 3-D GRE

> **Example**
> *DESS:*   *FFE, fat-saturated:*
> — TR = 25   — TR = 30–111
> — TE = 9   — TE = 20–27
> — Flip angle 35°   — Flip angle 15–25°

— Slab thickness: 50 mm (effective thickness approx. 0.9 mm)
— No. of partitions: 64
— Matrix: 512
— Saturation slab: axial (orthogonal) proximal to the slices (not for DESS)

Tips & Tricks
— If necessary immobilize forearm with sandbag

Modifications

Indirect Arthrography of the Wrist

(Investigation for tear in the ulnar triangular disc, lesion of the metacarpal ligaments, foreign body, tear in the wrist capsule)

Patient Preparation
— Intravenous injection of the contrast agent (Gd-DTPA 0.2 mmol/kg body weight)
— Have the patient go through intensive wrist exercises for 20–30 minutes and then run additional sequences

Sequences
Sequence 5 coronal (as sequence 1)

T1-weighted, fat-saturated

Example

SE, FS:	*GRE:*
— TR = 450–600	— TR = 400–600
— TE = 15–25	— TE = minimum (≤ 11)
or	— Flip angle 80–90°

or

SPIR

Example

— TR = 2200	— Flip angle 90°
— TE = 32	

— Slice thickness: 3 mm
— Slice gap: contiguous (factor 1.0)
— FOV: 120–150 mm
— Matrix: 512
— Saturation slab: axial (parallel) proximal to the slices and possibly

Sequence 6 axial

(as basic sequence 3, T1-weighted or fat-saturated)

or

Sequence 6 sagittal

T1-weighted, fat-saturated

Example

SE, FS:	*GRE:*
— TR = 450–600	— TR = 400–600
— TE = 15–25	— TE = minimum (≤ 11)
or	— Flip angle 80–90°

---

or

SPIR

Example

— TR = 2200	— Flip angle 90°
— TE = 32	

— Slice thickness: 3 mm
— Slice gap: 20 % of slice thickness ($\triangleq$ 0.6 mm or factor 1.2)
— FOV: 120–150 mm
— Matrix: 512
— Saturation slab: axial (parallel) proximal to the slices

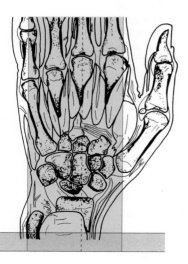

Wrist, sagittal,
sequence 6

Finger

Patient Preparation
— Have the patient go to the toilet before the study
— Explain the procedure to the patient
— Offer the patient ear protectors or ear plugs
— Ask the patient to undress above the waist except for underwear
— Ask the patient to remove anything containing metal (watch, jewelry, hearing aids, hairpins, body jewelry, etc.)

Positioning
— Prone: arm straight above the head, palm against the table; secure; surface coil
— Or supine: arm straight alongside the body

Sequences
— Scout: axial and sagittal (three planes, if possible)

Sequence 1 coronal (set up on sagittal slice)

TIRM or STIR

Example	
1.5 and 1.0 T:	*(1.0 and) 0.5 T:*
— TR = 5000–6500	— TR = 2200
— TE = 30–60	— TE = 30–60
— TI = 140	— TI = 100–130
— Flip angle 180°	— Flip angle 90°

or

T2-weighted, fat-saturated

Example
TSE, FS:
— TR = 2000–3500
— TE = 100

— Slice thickness: 3–4 mm
— Slice gap: contiguous ($\triangleq$ 0 mm or factor 1.0)
— FOV: 120–150 mm
— Saturation slab: axial proximal to the slices (across the distal forearm)

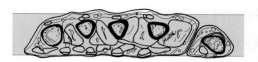

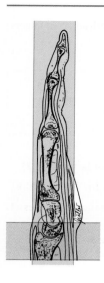

Finger, coronal, sequence 1

Sequence 2 coronal (as sequence 1)

T1-weighted

> **Example**
> — TR = 500–700
> — TE = 10–20

— Slice thickness: 3–4 mm
— Slice gap: 10% of slice thickness ($\triangleq$ 0.3–0.4 mm or factor 1.1)
— FOV: 120–150 mm
— Matrix: 512, if possible
— Saturation slab: axial proximal to the slices (across the distal forearm)

Sequence 3 sagittal (across the finger in question and both adjacent fingers)

T2-weighted

> **Example**
> *TSE:*
> — TR = 2000–4000
> — TE = 100–130

— Slice thickness: 3 mm
— Slice gap: 10–20% of slice thickness ($\triangleq$ 0.3–0.6 mm or factor 1.1–1.2)
— FOV: 120–150 mm
— Matrix: 512, if possible (NSA: about 4)
— Saturation slab: axial proximal to the slices for saturation of the vessels

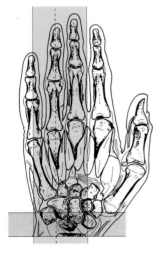

Finger, sagittal, sequence 3

Sequence 4 axial

T1-weighted

> **Example**
> — TR = 500–700
> — TE = 10–20

- Slice thickness: 3 mm
- Slice gap: 20–40% of slice thickness ($\triangleq$ 0.6–1.2 mm or factor 1.2–1.4)
- FOV: 120–150 mm
- Matrix: 512, if possible
- Saturation slab: axial proximal to the slices (across the distal forearm)

Tips & Tricks
- If necessary immobilize forearm with sandbag

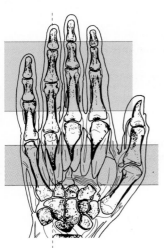

Finger, axial, sequence 4

Hip

Patient Preparation
— Have the patient go to the toilet before the study
— Explain the procedure to the patient
— Offer the patient ear protectors or ear plugs
— Have the patient undress except for underwear
— Ask the patient to remove anything containing metal (hearing aids, hairpins, body jewelry, etc.)

Positioning
— Supine
— Body array coil (body coil, wraparound coil)
— Cushion the legs with a small roll under the knees (do not elevate the thighs too much)
— Have the patient cross the arms over the upper abdomen

Sequences
— Scout: axial and coronal

Sequence 1 coronal across the femoral heads
(allow for an oblique presentation of the pelvis)

TIRM or STIR

Example	
1.5 and 1.0 T:	*(1.0 and) 0.5 T:*
— TR = 6500	— TR = 1800–2200
— TE = 30–60	— TE = 30–60
— TI = 140	— TI = 100–120
— Flip angle 180°	— Flip angle 90°

or

T2-weighted, fat-saturated

Example
TSE, FS:
— TR = 2000–3500
— TE = 100–120

— Slice thickness: 4 mm
— Slice gap: 20% of slice thickness ($\triangleq$ 0.8 mm or factor 1.2)
— FOV: 350–380 mm
— Saturation slab: axial superior to the slices for saturation of the vessels

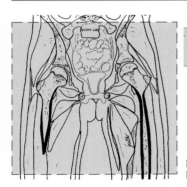
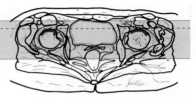

Hip, coronal across the femoral heads, sequence 1

Sequence 2 coronal across the femoral heads
(allow for an oblique presentation of the pelvis)

T1-weighted

> **Example**
> — TR = 450–600
> — TE = 12–25

— Slice thickness: 4–6 mm
— Slice gap: 20% of slice thickness ($\triangleq$ 0.8–1.2 mm or factor 1.2)
— Matrix: 512 (256)
— Saturation slab: axial superior to the slices for saturation of the vessels

Sequence 3 axial across the femoral heads and acetabula
(caudad to the lower aspect of the greater trochanter)

T2-weighted

> **Example**
> *TSE:*
> — TR = 2000–4000
> — TE = 100–130

— Slice thickness: 5–6 mm
— Slice gap: 20% of slice thickness ($\triangleq$ 1.0–1.2 mm or factor 1.2)
— FOV: approx. 350–380 mm (possibly rectangular FOV), adjust
— Saturation slab: axial (parallel) superior to the slices for saturation of the vessels

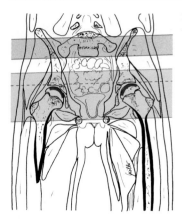

Hip, axial across the femoral heads and the acetabula, sequence 3

Sequence 4 sagittal across both femoral heads

T1-weighted

Example
— TR = 500–600
— TE = 10–12

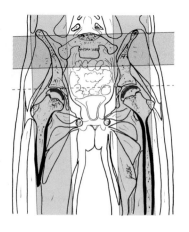

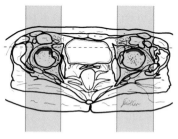

Hip, sagittal across both femoral heads, sequence 4

— Slice thickness: 5–6 mm
— Slice gap: 0–20% of slice thickness (≙ 0–1.2 mm or factor 0–1.2)
— FOV: approx. 380–400 mm
— Saturation slab: axial superior to the slices for saturation of the vessels

and possibly

Sequence 5 coronal across the femoral heads, as sequence 2 (T1-weighted) but after intravenous administration of contrast agent (e.g., Gd-DTPA), possibly with fat saturation

---

Tips & Tricks
— Positioning aid:
Center on anterior inferior iliac spine
— If the coronal images show vascular artifacts due to the iliac vessels, switching the phase encoding gradient to HF may help (with oversampling in order to avoid foldover)

Thigh

Patient Preparation
— Have the patient go to the toilet before the study
— Explain the procedure to the patient
— Offer the patient ear protectors or ear plugs
— Have the patient undress except for underwear
— Ask the patient to remove anything containing metal (hearing aids, hairpins, body jewelry, etc.)

Positioning

— Supine
— Body coil (body array coil, wraparound coil)
— Cushion the legs

Sequences
— Scout: all three planes

Sequence 1 coronal across both extremities (for comparison; *note:* allow for an oblique presentation) or else just the one under investigation

TIRM or STIR

Example	
1.5 and 1.0 T:	*(1.0 and) 0.5 T:*
— TR = 6500	— TR = 1600–2000
— TE = 14	— TE = 60
— TI = 140	— TI = 100–140
— Flip angle 180°	— Flip angle 90°

or

T2-weighted, fat-saturated

Example
TSE, FS:
— TR = 2000–3500
— TE = 90–100

— Slice thickness: 4–6 mm
— Slice gap: 20% of slice thickness ($\triangleq$ 0.8–1.2 mm or factor 1.2)
— FOV: 450–500 mm
— Saturation slab: axial superior to the slices for saturation of the vessels

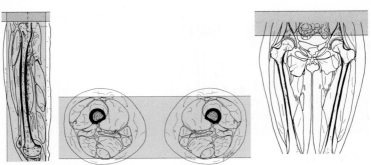

Thigh, coronal, sequence 1

Sequence 2 coronal across both extremities (for comparison; *note*: allow for an oblique presentation) or else just the one under investigation

T1-weighted

> **Example**
> — TR = 450–600
> — TE = 10–25

— Slice thickness: 4–6 mm
— Slice gap: 20% of slice thickness ($\triangleq$ 0.8–1.2 mm or factor 1.2)
— Saturation slab: axial superior to the slices for saturation of the vessels

Sequence 3 axial (the position of the slices depends on the pathologic findings or the purpose of the investigation)

T2-weighted

> **Example**
> *TSE:*
> — TR = 2000–4000
> — TE = 100–130

— Slice thickness: 6–8 mm
— Slice gap: 20–50% of slice thickness ($\triangleq$ 1.2–4 mm or factor 1.2–1.5)
— FOV: approx. 450–500 mm (when imaging only one thigh use approx. 200 mm)
— Saturation slab: axial (parallel) superior to the slices for saturation of the vessels

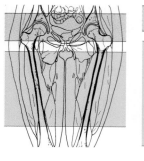
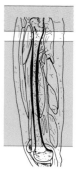

Thigh, axial, sequence 3

Sequence 4 sagittal (across the region in question)

T1-weighted

> **Example**
> — TR = 450–600
> — TE = 10–25

— Slice thickness: 6–8 mm
— Slice gap: 20% of slice thickness ($\triangleq$ 1.2–1.6 mm or factor 1.2)
— Phase encoding gradient: AP (or HF with oversampling)
— FOV: approx. 350–380 mm (possibly rectangular FOV, adjust)
— Saturation slab: no

and possibly

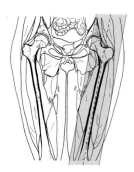
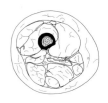
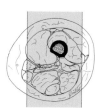

Thigh, sagittal,
sequence 4

Proton-density-weighted with spectral fat saturation

> **Example**
> *TSE:*
> — TR = 2000–2400
> — TE = 13–16
> — Flip angle 90°

- Slice thickness: 3 mm
- Slice gap: 20% of slice thickness (≙ 0.6 mm or factor 1.2)
- Phase encoding gradient: LR
- FOV: approx. 160 (–180) mm
- Saturation slab: axial (parallel) superior to the slices

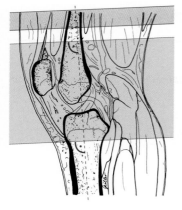

Knee, axial,
sequence 3

Sequence 4 coronal (or sagittal) (see above)

T1-weighted

> **Example**
> — TR = 450–600
> — TE = 15–25

- Slice thickness: 3–6 mm
- Slice gap: 20% of slice thickness (≙ 0.6–1.2 mm or factor 1.2)
- Saturation slab: axial superior to the slices

Tips & Tricks
— Cushion the knee well (sandbags, wedges)
— To avoid repeatedly having to set up two scout sequences (in the off-center position), have a right and left sagittal scout set up for the knee in the standard scout program; one scout always displays the joint while the other does not
— In children, comparative images of the two knees may be performed with the knees in the head coil. Secure the knees with cushions, and for the sequences either adjust TR according to the number of slices or run the sequences separately for each side
— The anterior cruciate ligament is delineated best at 15–20° of external rotation, the posterior cruciate ligament at 0° or 5° internal rotation

Modifications

Enhanced MRI of the Knee

(Investigation for, e.g., tumor, vascularization of an osteochondrosis dissecans lesion)

Patient Preparation
— Have intravenous line with extension set placed

Sequences

Sequence 1 coronal

TIRM or STIR (see basic sequence 1 above)
Sequence 2 sagittal, 3-D GRE (see basic sequence 2 above)

Sequence 3 coronal

T1-weighted

Example
— TR = 450–700
— TE = 12–25

— Slice thickness: 4–6 mm
— Slice gap: 20% of slice thickness ($\triangleq$ 0.8–1.2 mm or factor 1.2)
— Saturation slab: no

Sequence 4 (as sequence 3 but after administration of contrast agent – e.g., Gd-DTPA)

Sequence 5 axial (after contrast)

T1-weighted

> **Example**
> — TR = 450–700
> — TE = 12–25

— Slice thickness: 4–6 mm
— Slice gap: 20% of slice thickness ($\triangleq$ 0.8–1.2 mm or factor 1.2)
— Saturation slab: axial (parallel) superior to the slices

Indirect Arthrography

(Investigation for loose body, torn meniscus, injury of anterior cruciate ligament, or when noncontrast imaging was inconclusive)

Patient Preparation
— Intravenous administration of contrast agent (Gd-DTPA, 0.2 mmol/kg body weight)
— Have the patient move the knee intensively for 20–30 minutes

Sequences

Sequence 1 sagittal (slice position as in basic sequence 2)

T1-weighted, fat-saturated

> **Example**
> — TR = 450–700
> — TE = 12–25

or

GRE, fat-saturated

> **Example**
> — TR = 400–600
> — TE = minimum ($\leq$ 11)
> — Flip angle 80–90°

— Slice thickness: 3 mm
— Slice gap: 0–20% of slice thickness (≙ 0–0.6 mm or factor 1.2)
— Matrix: 512
— Saturation slab: axial superior to the slices

Sequence 2 coronal

T1-weighted, fat-saturated (see sequence 1)
— Slice thickness: 3–4 mm
— Slice gap: 20% of slice thickness (≙ 0.6–0.8 mm or factor 1.2)
— Saturation slab: axial superior to the slices

Sequence 3 axial

T1-weighted, fat-saturated (see sequence 1)
— Slice thickness: 3 mm
— Slice gap: 20% of slice thickness (≙ 0.6 mm or factor 1.2)
— Saturation slab: axial (parallel) superior to the slices

Sequence 4 coronal

TIRM or STIR or T2-weighted, fat-saturated (see basic sequence 1 above)

Lower Leg

Patient Preparation
— Have the patient go to the toilet before the study
— Explain the procedure to the patient
— Offer the patient ear protectors or ear plugs
— Ask the patient to undress except for underwear
— Ask the patient to remove anything containing metal (hearing aids, hairpins, body jewelry, etc.)
— If needed, have intravenous line placed

Positioning
— Supine
— Body array coil (wraparound coil, for children and small adults head/knee coil may also be possible)
— Internal rotation
— Cushion the legs

Sequences
— Scout: axial and sagittal

Sequence 1 coronal across one or both extremities (for comparison; *note:* allow for an oblique presentation)

TIRM or STIR

Example	
1.5 and 1.0 T:	*(1.0 and) 0.5 T:*
— TR = 6500	— TR = 1600–2000
— TE = 30–60	— TE = 60
— TI = 40	— TI = 100–140
— Flip angle 180°	— Flip angle 90°

or

T2-weighted, fat-saturated

Example	
TSE, FS:	— TE = 90–100
— TR = 2500–3500	

— Slice thickness: 4 mm
— Slice gap: 20% of slice thickness (≙ 0.8 mm or factor 1.2)
— FOV: approx. 400–450 mm
— Saturation slab: axial superior to the slices for saturation of the vessels

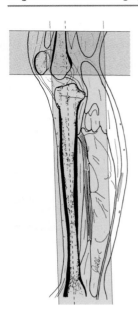
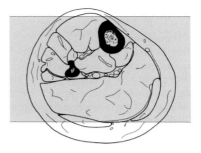

Lower leg, coronal,
sequence 1

Sequence 2 coronal across one or both extremities (for comparison;
note: allow for an oblique presentation)

T1-weighted

> **Example**
> — TR = 500–600
> — TE = 10–20

— Slice thickness: 4 mm
— Slice gap: 20% of slice thickness ($\triangleq$ 0.8 mm or factor 1.2)
— FOV: approx. 400–450 mm
— Matrix: 512, if possible
— Saturation slab: axial superior to the slices for saturation of the vessels

Sequence 3 axial

T2-weighted, possibly with fat saturation (slice position depending on the pathologic findings and/or the purpose of the investigation)

Example
TSE:
— TR = 2000–4000
— TE = 90–130

— Slice thickness: 5–6 mm
— Slice gap: 20–50 % of slice thickness ($\triangleq$ 1.0–3 mm or factor 1.2–1.5, depending on the question)
— FOV: approx. 380–400 mm for both lower legs or approx. 200 mm for just one
— Saturation slab: axial (parallel) superior to the slices for saturation of the vessels

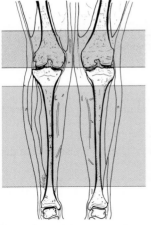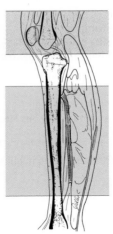

Lower leg, axial, sequence 3

Sequence 4 sagittal

T1-weighted

Example
— TR = 450–600
— TE = 10–25

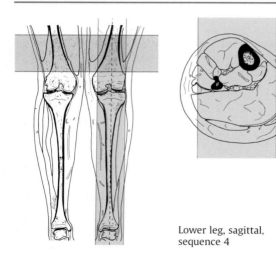

Lower leg, sagittal,
sequence 4

— Slice thickness: 4–6 mm
— Slice gap: 20% of slice thickness (≙ 0.8–1.2 mm or factor 1.2)
— FOV: approx. 380–400 mm (possibly rectangular FOV)
— Saturation slab: no

and possibly

Sequence 5 sagittal as sequence 4 but after administration of the contrast agent (e.g., Gd-DTPA i. v.)

Sequence 6 axial (across the region in question) after administration of the contrast agent

T1-weighted

> **Example**
> — TR = 450–600
> — TE = 10–25

— Slice thickness: 5–6 mm
— Slice gap: 20–50% of slice thickness (≙ 1.0–3 mm or factor 1.2–1.5, depending on the purpose of the investigation)
— FOV: approx. 400 mm for both lower legs or approx. 200 mm for just one
— Saturation slab: axial (parallel) superior to the slices for saturation of the vessels

Ankle

Patient Preparation
— Have the patient go to the toilet before the study
— Explain the procedure to the patient
— Offer the patient ear protectors or ear plugs
— Ask the patient to undress except for underwear
— Ask the patient to remove anything containing metal (hearing aids, hair-pins, body jewelry, watch etc.)

Positioning
— Supine
— Knee coil (head coil or wraparound coil for both ankles)
— Secure ankle in coil
— Cushion the other leg well

Sequences
— Scout: sagittal and axial (three planes, if possible)

Sequence 1 sagittal

TIRM or STIR

Example
1.5 and 1.0 T:
— TR = 6500
— TE = 30–60
— TI = 140
— Flip angle 180°

(1.0 and) 0.5 T:
STIR:
— TR = 1600–2200
— TE = 32
— TI = 100–130
— Flip angle 90°

or

T2-weighted, fat-saturated

Example
TSE, FS:
— TR = 2000–3500
— TE = 90–120

— Slice thickness: 3 mm
— Slice gap: 0–20 % of slice thickness ($\triangleq$ 0–0.6 mm or factor 1.0–1.2)
— FOV: large enough to include the toes, or use phase oversampling to avoid foldover of the toes, approx. 250 mm

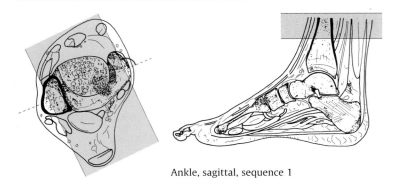

Ankle, sagittal, sequence 1

— Matrix: 512, if possible
— Saturation slab: axial superior to the slices

Sequence 2 coronal (= orthogonal to sequence 1)

T2-weighted, fat-saturated

Example
TSE, FS: *0.5 T:*
— TR = 2000–3500   *3-D FFE with fat saturation:*
— TE = 100–120   — TR = 30–110
                                        — TE = 20–27
                                        — Flip angle 15–25°

— Slice thickness: 3 mm
— Slice gap: 0–20% of slice thickness (≙ 0–0.6 mm or factor 1.0–1.2)
— FOV: approx. 160–180 mm

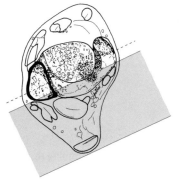

Ankle, coronal,
sequence 2

— Matrix: 512, if possible
— Saturation slab: no

Sequence 3 axial

T2-weighted

> **Example**
> *TSE:*
> — TR = 3000–4500
> — TE = 100–130

— Slice thickness: 4 mm
— Slice gap: 20% of slice thickness (≙ 0.8 mm or factor 1.2)
— Saturation slab: axial (parallel) superior to the slices

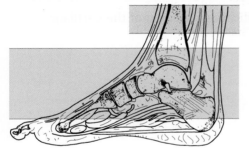

Ankle, axial, sequence 3

Sequence 4 coronal

T1-weighted

> **Example**
> — TR = 450–600
> — TE = 15–20
> — Flip angle 90°

— Slice thickness: 3 mm
— Slice gap: 10–20% of slice thickness (≙ 0.3–0.6 mm or factor 1.1–1.2)
— Saturation slab: no

Tips & Tricks

Optimized imaging of the
— Calcaneonavicular and deltoid ligaments (tibiocalcanean and talotibial part): coronal slice in maximum dorsiflexion (10–20°)
— Anterior and posterior talofibular ligaments: axial slice in maximum dorsiflexion (10–20°)
— Calcaneofibular ligament: axial slice in maximum plantar flexion (40–50°)
— Deltoid ligament (tibionavicular and anterior talotibial part): coronal slice in maximum plantar flexion (40–50°)

Modifications

Technical Study Modification: Imaging of the Cartilage
(Possibly as an additional study)

Sequence 5 sagittal

GRE, fat-saturated

Example
1.5 and 1.0 T:
FLASH-3-D FS:
— TR = 770
— TE = 11
— Flip angle 60°

Indirect Arthrography of the Ankle
(Investigation for loose body, capsular tear, ligament lesion, cartilage damage, if noncontrast study was inconclusive)

Patient Preparation
— Administration of contrast agent (Gd-DTPA 0.2 mmol/kg body weight i. v.)
— Have the patient move the ankle intensively for 20–30 minutes and then run additional sequences

Sequences

Sequence 1 sagittal

T1-weighted, fat-saturated (same slice position as for basic sequence 1 above)

> **Example**
> — TR = 450–600
> — TE = 15–25

or

GRE, fat-saturated

> **Example**
> — TR = 400–600
> — TE = minimum ($\leq$–11)
> — Flip angle 80–90°

— Slice thickness: 2–3 mm
— Slice gap: 10–20% of slice thickness ($\triangleq$ 0.2–0.6 mm or factor 1.1–1.2)
— Phase encoding gradient: PA with 50% oversampling (or: HF with 100% oversampling)
— Matrix: 512
— Saturation slab: axial (parallel) superior to the slices

Sequence 2 coronal

T1-weighted, fat-saturated (same slice position as for basic sequence 2 above)

> **Example**
> — TR = 450–600
> — TE = 15–25

or

GRE, fat-saturated

> **Example**
> — TR = 400–600
> — TE = minimum ($\leq$ 11)
> — Flip angle 80–90°

— Slice thickness: 2–3 mm
— Slice gap: 20% of slice thickness ($\triangleq$ 0.4–0.6 mm or factor 1.2)
— Phase encoding gradient: RL

— Matrix: 512
— FOV: approx. 160 mm (possibly rectangular FOV)
— Saturation slab: axial superior to the slices

Sequence 3 axial

T1-weighted, fat-saturated (same slice position as for basic sequence 3 above)

> **Example**
> — TR = 450–600
> — TE = 15–25

or

GRE, fat-saturated

> **Example**
> — TR = 400–600
> — TE = minimum ($\triangleq$ 11)
> — Flip angle 80–90°

— Slice thickness: 3 mm
— Slice gap: 20% of slice thickness ($\triangleq$ 0.6 mm or factor 1.2)
— Phase encoding gradient: RL
— Matrix: 512
— Saturation slab: axial (parallel) superior to the slices

MRI of the Achilles Tendon

Sequences

Sequence 1 sagittal

TIRM or STIR (as basic sequence 1 above)

Sequence 2 sagittal

T1-weighted

> **Example**
> — TR = 450–600
> — TE = 15–25

— Slice thickness: 3 mm
— Slice gap: 10–20% of slice thickness ($\triangleq$ 0.3–0.6 mm or factor 1.1–1.2)
— Phase encoding gradient: PA with 50% oversampling
— Saturation slab: axial superior to the slices and coronal across the forefoot

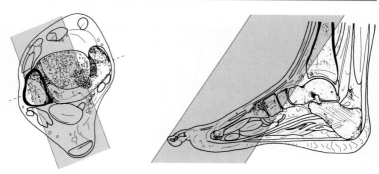

Achilles tendon, sagittal, sequence 2

Sequence 3 paracoronal across the Achilles tendon

T2-weighted, fat-saturated (as basic sequence 2)

and possibly

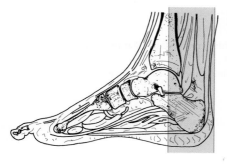

Achilles tendon, paracoronal, sequence 3

Sequence 4 axial

T1-weighted, fat-saturated, after administration of contrast agent (e.g., Gd-DTPA)

Example
— TR = 450–600
— TE = 15–25

or

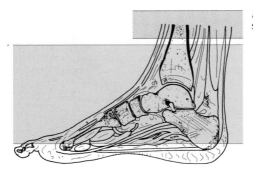

Achilles tendon, axial, sequence 4

SPIR

Example
— TR = 1700–2200
— TE = 15–32
— Flip angle 90°

— Slice thickness: 3 mm
— Slice gap: 20–40% of slice thickness ($\triangleq$ 0.6–1.2 mm or factor 1.2–1.4)
— Phase encoding gradient: RL
— Saturation slab: axial (parallel) superior to the slices

Sequence 5 sagittal

T1-weighted (as sequence 2 but after administration of contrast agent)

Enhanced MRI of the Ankle
(Investigation for, e.g., tumor, vascularization of an osteochondrosis dissecans lesion)

Patient Preparation
— Have intravenous line with extension set placed

Sequences

Sequence 1 sagittal

TIRM or STIR (as basic sequence 1 above)

Sequence 2 coronal

T2-weighted, fat-saturated (as basic sequence 2 above)

Sequence 3 coronal

T1-weighted, fat-saturated

> **Example**
> — TR = 450–700
> — TE = 12–25

— Slice thickness: 6 mm
— Slice gap: 20 % of slice thickness ($\triangleq$ 1.2 mm or factor 1.2)
— Saturation slab: no

Sequence 4 as sequence 3 but after administration of contrast agent (e.g., Gd-DTPA 0.1–0.2 mmol/kg body weight)

Sequence 5 axial

T1-weighted, fat-saturated

> **Example**
> — TR = 450–700
> — TE = 12–25

— Slice thickness: 4–6 mm
— Slice gap: 20 % of slice thickness ($\triangleq$ 0.8–1.2 mm or factor 1.2)
— Saturation slab: axial (parallel) superior to the slices

Forefoot

Patient Preparation
— Have the patient go to the toilet before the study
— Explain the procedure to the patient
— Offer the patient ear protectors or ear plugs
— Ask the patient to undress except for underwear
— Ask the patient to remove anything containing metal (hearing aids, hair-pins, body jewelry, watch, etc.)

Positioning

— Supine: secure foot in coil (e.g., head coil, bring sole into the vertical and rest against some foam rubber, or wraparound coil), cushion the other leg
— Or prone: back of the foot flat against the table (e.g., in knee coil for improved signal-to-noise ratio)

Sequences
— Scout: three planes

Sequence 1 axial (= coronal with respect to the foot; adjusted for the oblique course of the metatarsals)

TIRM or STIR

Example

1.5 and 1.0 T:
— TR = 6500
— TE = 30–60
— TI = 140
— Flip angle 180°

(1.0 and) 0.5 T:
STIR:
— TR = 1600–2200
— TE = 30–60
— TI = 100–140
— Flip angle 90°

---

or

T2-weighted, fat-saturated

Example
TSE, FS:
— TR = 2000–3500
— TE = 100–120

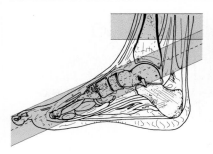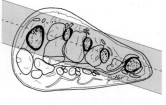

Forefoot, axial, sequence 1

— Slice thickness: 3 mm
— Slice gap: 10–20 % of slice thickness (≙ 0.3–0.6 mm or factor 1.1–1.2)
— Saturation slab: axial superior to the slices

Sequence 2 axial (as basic sequence 1 above)

T1-weighted

> **Example**
> — TR = 450–600
> — TE = 15–25

— Slice thickness: 4 mm
— Slice gap: 10 % of slice thickness (≙ 0.4 mm or factor 1.1)
— Saturation slab: no

Sequence 3 coronal (orthogonal to sequence 1 = axial with respect to the foot)

T2-weighted, fat-saturated

> **Example**
> *TSE, FS:*   *3-D FFE with fat saturation:*
> — TR = 2000–3500   — TR = 30–110
> — TE = 100–120   — TE = 20–27
>   — Flip angle 15–25°

— Slice thickness: 3 mm
— Slice gap: 10 % of slice thickness (≙ 0.3 mm or factor 1.1)
— Saturation slab: axial (possibly oblique) superior to the slices

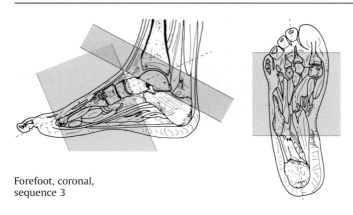

Forefoot, coronal,
sequence 3

Sequence 4 sagittal

T2-weighted

> **Example**
> *TSE:*
> — TR = 2500–4000
> — TE = 90–120

— Slice thickness: 4 mm
— Slice gap: 10–20% of slice thickness ($\triangleq$ 0.4–0.8 mm or factor 1.1–1.2)
— Saturation slab: axial superior to the slices

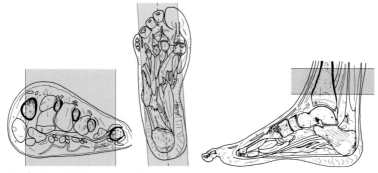

Forefoot, sagittal, sequence 4

Modifications

Enhanced MRI of the Forefoot

(Investigation for, e.g., tumor, vascularization of osteonecrosis or osteomyelitis)

Patient Preparation
— Have intravenous line with extension set placed

Sequences

Sequence 1 axial

TIRM or STIR (as basic sequence 1 above)

Sequence 2 axial

T1-weighted (as basic sequence 2 above)

Sequence 3 coronal

T2-weighted, fat-saturated (as basic sequence 3 above)
Administration of contrast agent (e.g., Gd-DTPA 0.1–0.2 mmol/kg body weight i. v.)

Sequence 4 axial

T1-weighted, as basic sequence 2 but after administration of contrast agent

Sequence 5 coronal

T1-weighted, as basic sequence 2 but after administration of contrast agent (with fat saturation, if needed), slice position as for sequence 3

Magnetic Resonance Imaging:
Spine

Cervical Spine

Patient Preparation
— Have the patient go to the toilet before the study
— Explain the procedure to the patient; in particular, ask the patient to keep swallowing and movement to a minimum (a comfortable position without pain is important) so as to avoid artifacts
— Offer the patient ear protectors or ear plugs
— Ask the patient to remove anything containing metal (dentures, hearing aids, hairpins, body jewelry, etc.)
— If needed, have an intravenous line placed (investigation for, e.g., tumor, multiple sclerosis, spondylodiskitis, abscess)

> **Positioning**
>
> — Supine on cervical spine coil
> — Cushion the legs
> — Arms straight alongside the body (cushion them, if needed)

Sequences
— Scout: sagittal and coronal (three planes, if possible)

Sequence 1 sagittal (plot on coronal scout; as many slices as needed to delineate all of the spine)

T2-weighted

> **Example**
> *TSE:*
> — TR = 2500–4000
> — TE = 100–120

— Slice thickness: 3–4 mm
— Slice gap: 20% of slice thickness ($\triangleq$ 0.6–0.8 mm or factor 1.2)
— Phase encoding gradient: HF with 100% oversampling because of foldover, flow compensation (CSF; alternatively, instead of flow compensation: large turbo factor, e.g.,15–25, and several NSAs)
— FOV: approx. 240–260 mm
— Saturation slab: coronal anterior to the vertebrae

Sequence 2 sagittal (as sequence 1)

Proton-density-weighted

> **Example**
> *TSE:*
> — TR = 1200–2000
> — TE = 12–20

or

T1-weighted

> **Example**
> *TSE:*
> — TR = 450–600
> — TE = 12–25

— Slice thickness: 3–4 mm
— Slice gap: 20% of slice thickness ($\triangleq$ 0.6–0.8 mm or factor 1.2)
— Phase encoding gradient: AP
— Saturation slab:
   - Coronal anterior (and possibly posterior) to the spine
   - Possibly axial superior to the sagittal slices
   - Possibly axial inferior to the sagittal slices

or

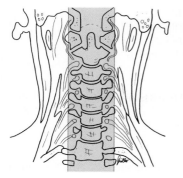 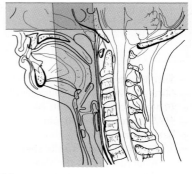

Cervical spine, sagittal, sequences 1 and 2
(with additional axial saturation slab)

Sequences 1 and 2 sagittal, double echo

T2 and proton-density-weighted

> **Example**
> — TR = 2000
> — TE = shortest (e.g., 20–30/120)
>   Otherwise as sequence 1

Sequence 3 axial parallel to the relevant vertebral end plates (for a normal cervical spine continuous slices from, e.g., C4 to T1 are enough)

Proton-density-weighted

> **Example**
> *TSE:*
> — TR = 1700
> — TE = 12

or

T2-weighted

> **Example**
> *GRE:*
> *1.5 (and 1.0) T:*   *1.0 (and 1.5) T:*
> — TR = 850   — TR = 500
> — TE = 26   — TE = 18
> — Flip angle 30°   — Flip angle 20°
>   *0.5 T:*
>   — TR = 55
>   — TE = 27
>   — Flip angle 6°

- Slice thickness: 3–4 mm
- Slice gap: 20% of slice thickness (≙ 0.6–0.8 mm or factor 1.2)
- Phase encoding gradient: PA
- FOV: approx. 180–200 mm
- Saturation slab:
  - Coronal anterior to the spine
  - Axial (parallel to the slices) superior to the slice slab (this saturation slab is not applicable for motion artifact suppression)
  - Axial (parallel to the slices) inferior to the slice slab (this saturation slab is not applicable for motion artifact suppression)

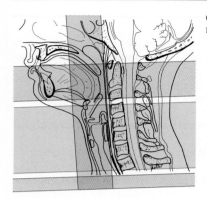

Cervical spine, axial, parallel to the relevant end plates, sequence 3

Sequence 4 coronal

T2-weighted

> **Example**
> *TSE (with larger turbo factor, e.g., 20):*
> — TR = 3000–4000
> — TE = 100–140

— Slice thickness: 4–6 mm
— Slice gap: 10 % of slice thickness ($\triangleq$ 0.4–0.6 mm or factor 1.1)
— Phase encoding gradient: LR
— Saturation slab: no

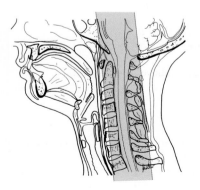

Cervical spine, coronal, sequence 4

Tips & Tricks
— In patients with increased kyphosis cushion the pelvis; in patients with cervical spine problems it may be advisable to elevate the head somewhat and cushion it
— Cushion the neck
— If needed, have the patient put on a neck brace (under the coil, secures the neck and ensures stability)
— Before running sequence 1, have the patient swallow and clear his/her throat
— In patients with severe scoliosis ensure that enough slices capture the lateral aspects
— In patients with a short neck the upper part of the cervical spine coil may not fit: either use phased-array coil or acquire the images without the upper strap (image quality will be poorer); for phased-array coil select cervical and thoracic
— Positioning aids:
Cervical spine: center on the middle of the throat (lower in patients with a short neck—almost all the way to the jugular fossa)

Modifications

Suspected Tumor, Suspected Spondylodiskitis, Abscess

Patient Preparation
— Have intravenous line with extension set placed

Sequences

Sequence 1 sagittal

T2-weighted (as basic sequence 1 above)

Sequence 2 sagittal (as basic sequence 2 above, T1-weighted)

Sequence 3 axial (across the region in question)

T1-weighted

> **Example**
> *TSE:*
> — TR = 500–650
> — TE = 12–25

- Slice thickness: 4 mm
- Slice gap: 20 % of slice thickness (≙ 0.8 mm or factor 1.2)
- FOV: approx. 180–200 mm
- Three saturation slabs:
  - Orthogonal (coronal) to the slices, slab saturates the region anterior to the spine
  - Axial (parallel to the slices) superior to the slice slab (not applicable for motion artifact suppression)
  - Axial (parallel to the slices) inferior to the slice slab (not applicable for motion artifact suppression)

Sequence 4 axial

T1-weighted as sequence 3, but after administration of contrast agent (e.g., Gd-DTPA)

Sequence 5 sagittal

T1-weighted as sequence 2, but after administration of contrast agent (e.g., Gd-DTPA)

Suspected Disseminated Encephalomyelitis or Syringomyelia

Patient Preparation
— Have intravenous line with extension placed

Sequences
Sequence 1 sagittal

T2-weighted (as basic sequence 1 above)

Sequence 2 axial (across the region in question)

T2-weighted

Example

TSE:	*1.0 (and 1.5) T:*
— TR = 3000–4500	— TR = 500
— TE = 100–130	— TE = 18
GRE:	— Flip angle 20°
1.5 (and 1.0) T:	*1.0 and 0.5 T:*
— TR = 850	— TR = 55
— TE = 26	— TE = 20–27
— Flip angle 30°	— Flip angle 5–6°

— Slice thickness, slice gap, and saturation slab: as basic sequence 3 above

Sequence 3 sagittal (as basic sequence 2 above, T1-weighted)

Sequence 4 sagittal (as basic sequence 2 above, T1-weighted, but after administration of contrast agent, e.g., Gd-DTPA)

Trauma, Suspected Fracture

Patient Preparation
— If needed, have intravenous line with extension set placed

Sequences

Sequence 1 sagittal

TIRM or STIR

> **Example**
> — TR = 6500   or
> — TE = 30–60   — TR = 1400–1600
> — TI = 140   — TE = 15
> — Flip angle 180° — TI = 100–120

or

T2-weighted, fat-saturated

> **Example**
> *TSE, FS:*
> — TR = 3000–3500
> — TE = 100–120

— Slice thickness: 3–4 mm
— Slice gap: 10–20% of slice thickness ($\triangleq$ 0.3–0.8 mm or factor 1.1–1.2)
— Phase encoding gradient: AP, flow compensation (alternatively: HF, large turbo factor, e.g., 15–25, multiple NSAs, 100% oversampling)
— Saturation slab:
  - Orthogonal to the slices, slab saturates the region anterior to the spine
  - Axial superior to the slices (decreases CSF pulsation)

Sequence 2 sagittal (as basic sequence 2, T1-weighted)

T1-weighted

> **Example**
> *TSE:*
> — TR = 450–600
> — TE = 12–25

— Slice thickness, slice gap, and saturation slab: as basic sequence 1 above

Sequence 3 axial (across the region in question)

T2-weighted

Example	
GRE:	*1.0 and 0.5 T:*
1.5 and 1.0 T:	— TR = 55
— TR = 850	— TE = 20–27
— TE = 26	— Flip angle 5–6°
— Flip angle 30°	
or	
— TR = 500	
— TE = 18	
— Flip angle 20°	

- Slice thickness: 4 mm
- Slice gap: 20% of slice thickness (≙ 0.8 mm or factor 1.2)
- Three saturation slabs:
  - Orthogonal (coronal) to the slices, slab saturates the region anterior to the spine
  - Axial superior to the slices
    (not applicable for motion artifact suppression)
  - Perhaps axial inferior to the slices
    (not applicable for motion artifact suppression)

Sequence 4 coronal (as basic sequence 4 above)

possibly

Sequence 5 sagittal

T1-weighted (as basic sequence 2 above, but after administration of contrast agent)

Sequence 6 axial (across the region in question, as basic sequence 3 above, but after administration of contrast agent)

T1-weighted

Example
TSE:
— TR = 500–700
— TE = 12–25

Thoracic Spine

Patient Preparation
— Have the patient go to the toilet before the study
— Explain the procedure to the patient, in particular in relation to avoiding motion artifacts (a comfortable position without pain is important)
— Offer the patient ear protectors or ear plugs
— Ask the patient to remove anything containing metal (hearing aids, hairpins, necklaces, bra, body jewelry, etc.)
— If needed, have intravenous line placed (investigation for, e.g., tumor, multiple sclerosis, spondylodiskitis, abscess)

Positioning
— Supine
— Cushion the legs and secure them if necessary
— The arms should be alongside the body except in obese patients, where they should be raised above the head
— Positioning aid:
Center on a spot about 2–3 inches (5–8 cm) below the jugular fossa (or on the center of the sternum)

Sequences
— Scout: sagittal and coronal (three planes, if possible)
Note: Long sagittal scout (FOV approx. 500 mm) to count the vertebrae (perhaps use full-body coil)

Sequence 1 sagittal (plot on coronal scout, as many slices as needed to acquire all of the spine)

T2-weighted

Example
TSE:
— TR = 3000–3500
— TE = 100–120

— Slice thickness: 4 mm
— Phase encoding gradient: PA, flow compensation (or FH, but then with 100% oversampling, select TSE sequence with large turbo factor, e.g., 15–25, and run several NSAs in order to minimize flow artifacts)
— FOV: approx. 300–350 mm
— Matrix: 512

— Saturation slab:
  - Coronal, slab saturates the region anterior to the spine (aorta, intestines, breathing artifacts)
  - Possibly coronal for saturation of the dorsal fatty tissue

Sequence 2 sagittal (as basic sequence 1 above)

Proton-density-weighted

> **Example**
> *TSE:*
> — TR = 1200–2000
> — TE = 12–20

or

T1-weighted

> **Example**
> *TSE:*
> — TR = 500–750
> — TE = 12–25

— Phase encoding gradient: PA, flow compensation (or FH, but then with 100 % oversampling, large turbo factor, e.g., 15–25, multiple NSAs)
— Slice thickness, slice gap, and saturation slab: as basic sequence 1 above

or

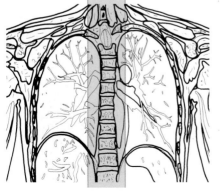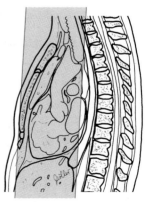

Thoracic spine, sagittal, sequences 1 and 2

Sequences 1 and 2 sagittal, double echo

T2/proton-density-weighted (otherwise as basic sequence 1 above)

Sequence 3 axial parallel to the corresponding end plates either continuous or (for severe kyphosis) adjust each segment individually (for severe scoliosis on coronal scout also adjust laterally to the end plates)

Proton-density-weighted

> **Example**
> — TSE = 1500–2000
> — TE = 12–25

or

T2-weighted

> **Example**
> *GRE:*   *0.5 T:*
> *1.5 and 1.0 T:*   — TR = 55
> — TR = 850   — TE = 27
> — TE = 26   — Flip angle 6°
> — Flip angle 30°
> or
> — TR = 500
> — TE = 18
> — Flip angle 20°

— Slice thickness: 3–4 mm
— Slice gap: 0–20% of slice thickness ($\triangleq$ 0–0.8 mm or factor 1.0–1.2)
— FOV: approx. 180–200 mm
— Saturation slab: orthogonal (coronal) to the slices, slab saturates the region anterior to the spine

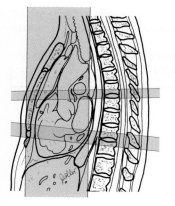 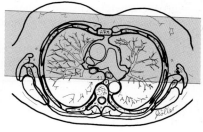

Thoracic spine, axial to the relevant end plates, sequence 3

Sequence 4 coronal

T2-weighted

> **Example**
> *TSE with larger turbo factor (e.g., 20):*
> — TR = 3000–4000
> — TE = 90–140

— Slice thickness: 6 mm
— Slice gap: 10–20 % of slice thickness (≙ 0.6–1.2 mm or factor 1.1–1.2)
— Saturation slab: no

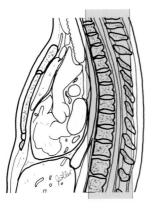
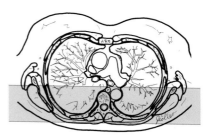

Thoracic spine, axial to the relevant
end plates, sequence 4

Tips & Tricks
— In patients with increased kyphosis cushion the back; in those with additional neck complaints it may be advisable to elevate and cushion the head
— In patients with severe scoliosis, ensure that in the sagittal images enough slices capture the lateral aspects

Modifications

Suspected Tumor or Spondylodiskitis, Abscess

Patient Preparation
— Have intravenous line with extension set placed

Sequences

Sequence 1 (see above)

Sequence 2 sagittal (as basic sequence 2 above, T1-weighted)

Sequence 3 axial (across the region in question; in the case of severe scoliosis also adjust on coronal scout; *note:* for metastases also image the vertebra immediately above and below the one in question)

T1-weighted

> **Example**
> *TSE:*
> — TR = 500–700
> — TE = 12–25

— Slice thickness: 4 mm
— Slice gap: 20 % of slice thickness ($\triangleq$ 0.8 mm or factor 1.2)
— Saturation slab: orthogonal (coronal) to the slices, slab saturates region anterior to the spine

Sequence 4 axial

T1-weighted (as basic sequence 3 above, but after administration of contrast agent, e.g., Gd-DTPA)

Sequence 5 sagittal

T1-weighted (as basic sequence 2, but after administration of contrast agent)

Trauma, Suspected Fracture

Patient Preparation
— If necessary, have intravenous line with extension set placed

Sequences
Sequence 1 sagittal

TIRM or STIR

Example	
— TR = 6500	— TI = 140
— TE = 30–60	— Flip angle 180°

or

T2-weighted, fat-saturated

Example
TSE, FS:
— TR = 3000–4500
— TE = 80–120

— Slice thickness: 4 mm
— Slice gap: 20% of slice thickness (≙ 0.8 mm or factor 1.2)
— Phase encoding gradient: AP, flow compensation (alternatively FH, large turbo factor, e.g., for STIR 9–15 and for TSE 15–25, multiple NSAs, 100% oversampling)
— Three saturation slabs:
  - Orthogonal to the slices, slab saturates the region anterior to the spine
  - Possibly axial superior to the sagittal slices
  - Possibly axial inferior to the sagittal slices

Sequence 2 sagittal (as basic sequence 2 above, T1-weighted)

Sequence 3 axial (across the region in question, for severe scoliosis also adjust on coronal scout; as basic sequence 3 above, T2-weighted)

Sequence 4 coronal (as basic sequence 4 above)

possibly

Sequence 5 sagittal

T1-weighted, fat-saturated, otherwise as sequence 2 but after intravenous administration of contrast agent (e.g., Gd-DTPA)

Sequence 6 axial

T1-weighted (across the region in question) after administration of contrast agent

---

Example
TSE:
— TR = 500–700
— TE = 12–25

- Slice thickness: 4 mm
- Slice gap: 20 % of slice thickness ($\triangleq$ 0.8 mm or factor 1.2)
- Saturation slab: orthogonal (coronal) to the slices, slab saturates the region anterior to the spine

Lumbar Spine

Patient Preparation
— Have the patient go to the toilet; the bladder must be empty
— Explain the procedure to the patient, in particular with a view to avoiding motion artifacts (a comfortable position without pain is important)
— Offer the patient ear protectors or ear plugs
— Ask the patient to remove anything containing metal (hearing aids, hairpins, pants, belt, bra, body jewelry, etc.)
— If necessary, have intravenous line placed (e.g., if the investigation is for tumor, multiple sclerosis, spondylodiskitis, or abscess)

Positioning
— Supine
— Spine coil
— Cushion the legs and secure them if needed
— Arms alongside the body (over the head for obese patients)

Sequences
— Scout: sagittal and coronal (three planes, if possible)

Sequence 1 sagittal (plot on coronal scout, as many slices as needed to image the whole spine)

T2-weighted

Example
TSE:
— TR = 3000–3500
— TE = 100–120

— Slice thickness: 4 mm
— Slice gap: 20% of slice thickness ($\triangleq$ 0.8 mm or factor 1.2)
— Phase encoding gradient: FH with 100% oversampling
— FOV: approx. 320–350 mm
— Matrix: 512
— Saturation slab: coronal, slab saturates the region anterior to the spine (aorta, intestines, breathing artifacts)

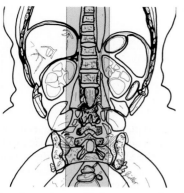 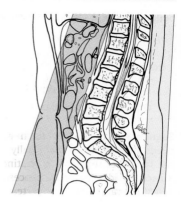

Lumbar spine, sagittal, sequences 1 and 2

Sequence 2 sagittal (as sequence 1 above)

Proton-density-weighted

> **Example**
> *TSE:*
> — TR = 1500–2500
> — TE = 12–20

or

T1-weighted

> **Example**
> *SE:*
> — TR = 450–600
> — TE = 12–25

— Slice thickness: 4 mm
— Slice gap: 20 % of slice thickness ($\triangleq$ 0.8 mm or factor 1.2)
— Phase encoding gradient: AP, flow compensation (or FH with 100 % over-sampling)
    saturation slab:
    • Coronal, slab saturates region anterior to the spine (aorta, intestines, breathing artifacts)
    • Perhaps coronal, saturation of the dorsal fatty tissue
or

Sequences 1 + 2 sagittal, double echo

T2/proton-density-weighted

> **Example**
> — TR = 2000–3000
> — TE = shortest (120)
> — Otherwise as sequence 1

Sequence 3 axial parallel to the relevant end plates (usually each segment needs to be adjusted individually; if no abnormalities are found, imaging of the last three segments is routine; *note:* keep slice overlap on the dorsal aspect outside the spinous processes, if possible; in cases of severe scoliosis, adjust laterally to the end plates on the coronal scout as well)

Proton-density-weighted

> **Example**
> *TSE:*
> — TR = 1700
> — TE = 12

or

T2-weighted

> **Example**
> *GRE:*   *0.5 T:*
> *1.5 and 1.0 T:*   — TR = 55
> — TR = 850   — TE = 27
> — TE = 26   — Flip angle 6°
> — Flip angle 30°
> or
> — TR = 500
> — TE = 18
> — Flip angle 20°

— Slice thickness: 3–4 mm
— Slice gap: 0–20 % of slice thickness ($\triangleq$ 0–0.8 mm or factor 1.0–1.2)
— FOV: 180–200 mm
— Saturation slab: orthogonal (coronal) to the slices, slab saturates the region anterior to the spine

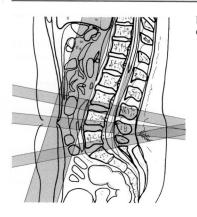

Lumbar spine, axial—parallel to the end plates, sequence 3

Sequence 4 coronal

T2-weighted

> **Example**
> *TSE with larger turbo factor (e.g., 20):*
> — TR = 3000
> — TE = 140

— Slice thickness: 6 mm
— Slice gap: 10–20 % of slice thickness ($\triangleq$ 0.6–1.2 mm or factor 1.1–1.2)
— Phase encoding gradient: LR
— Saturation slab: no

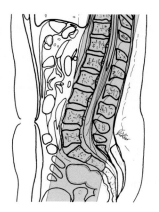

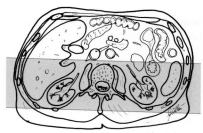

Lumbar spine, coronal, sequence 4

> **Tips & Tricks**
> — In patients with increased kyphosis; cushion the back; in those with additional neck complaints it may be advisable to elevate and cushion the head
> — If the patient is in pain, secure cushions to the outside of the knees with straps (this relaxes the back muscles)
> — In patients with severe scoliosis, ensure that enough slices will capture the lateral aspects
> — Positioning aid:
>   Center on a spot about 2–3 inches (5–8 cm) above the superior anterior iliac spine or iliac crest (in a tall patient)

Modifications

After Lumbar Disk Surgery

Patient Preparation
— Have intravenous line with extension set placed

Sequences

Sequence 1 sagittal

T2-weighted (as basic sequence 1 above)

Sequence 2 sagittal

Proton-density-weighted (as basic sequence 2 above)

Sequence 3 axial (parallel to the end plates; in cases of severe scoliosis adjust on coronal scout as well)

T1-weighted

Example
TSE:
— TR = 450–650
— TE = 12–25

— Slice thickness: 4 mm
— Slice gap: 0–20% of slice thickness ($\triangle$ 0–0.8 mm or factor 1.0–1.2)
— FOV: approx. 180–200 mm

— Saturation slab:
  - Orthogonal (coronal) to the slices, slab saturates the region anterior to the spine
  - Possibly axial (parallel to the slices) superior to the slice slab
  - Possibly axial (parallel to the slices) inferior to the slice slab

Sequence 4 axial (as sequence 3, but after administration of contrast agent, e.g., Gd-DTPA)

and possibly

Sequence 5 sagittal

(as basic sequence 2, T1-weighted, but after administration of contrast agent)

Suspected Tumor or Spondylodiskitis, Abscess

Patient Preparation
— Have intravenous line with extension set placed

Sequences

Sequence 1 sagittal (see above)

Sequence 2 sagittal (as basic sequence 2, T1-weighted)

Sequence 3 axial (across the region in question)

T1-weighted

> **Example**
> *TSE:*
> — TR = 500–700
> — TE = 12–25

— Slice thickness: 4 mm
— Slice gap: 0–20% of slice thickness (≙ 0–0.8 mm or factor 1.0–1.2)
— FOV: 180–200 mm
— Saturation slab: orthogonal (coronal) to the slices; slab saturates the region anterior to the spine

Sequence 4 axial

T1-weighted, as sequence 3, but after administration of contrast agent

Sequence 5 sagittal

T1-weighted, as sequence 2, but after administration of contrast agent (e.g., Gd-DTPA)

Trauma, Suspected Fracture

Patient Preparation
— If necessary, have intravenous line with extension set placed

Sequences

Sequence 1 sagittal (slice position as for basic sequence 1)

TIRM or STIR

Example	
— TR = 6500	— TI = 140
— TE = 30–60	— Flip angle 180°

or

T2-weighted, fat-saturated

Example
TSE, FS:
— TR = 3000–4000
— TE = 80–120

— Slice thickness: 4 mm
— Slice gap: 0–20 % of slice thickness ($\triangleq$ 0–0.8 mm or factor 1.0–1.2)
— Phase encoding gradient: PA, flow compensation (or FH, but in that case with 100 % oversampling)
— Matrix: 256
— Saturation slab:
  ● Orthogonal to the slices, slab saturates the region anterior to the spine
  ● Perhaps axial superior to the sagittal slices
  ● Perhaps axial inferior to the sagittal slices

Sequence 2 sagittal (as basic sequence 2, T1-weighted)

Sequence 3 axial (across the region in question)

T2-weighted

> **Example**
> *GRE:*   *0.5 T:*
> *1.5 and 1.0 T:*   — TR = 55
> — TR = 850   — TE = 27
> — TE = 26   — Flip angle 6°
> — Flip angle 30°
> or
> — TR = 500
> — TE = 18
> — Flip angle 20°

Sequence 4 coronal (as basic sequence 4)

T2-weighted

> **Example**
> *TSE with larger turbo factor (e.g., 20):*
> — TR = 3000–4000
> — TE = 100–140

— Slice thickness: 6 mm
— Slice gap: 10–20% of slice thickness ($\triangleq$ 0.6–1.2 mm or factor 1.1–1.2)
— Saturation slab: no

and possibly

Sequence 5 sagittal

T1-weighted (as sequence 5, but after administration of contrast agent, e.g., Gd-DTPA)

Sequence 6 axial (across the region in question)

T1-weighted

> **Example**
> *TSE:*
> — TR = 500–700
> — TE = 12–25

— Slice thickness: 4 mm
— Slice gap: 0–20% of slice thickness ($\triangleq$ 0–0.8 mm or factor 1.0–1.2)
— Saturation slab: orthogonal (coronal) to the slices, slab saturates the region anterior to the spine

Sacroiliac Joints

Sequences

Sequence 1 sagittal

T2-weighted

Example
— TR = 2000–3500
— TE = 100–130

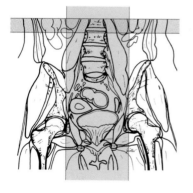
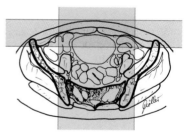
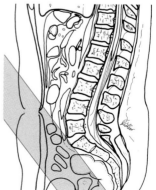

Sacroiliac joints, sagittal,
sequence 1

— Slice thickness: 5 mm
— Slice gap: 10–20% of slice thickness ($\triangleq$ 0.5–1.0 mm or factor 1.1–1.2)
— FOV: approx. 240–250 mm
— Matrix: 512
— Saturation slab:
  - Axial, superior to the slices for saturation of the vessels
  - Paracoronal, ventral to the subcutaneous fat and the intestines

Sequence 2 para-axial

T2-weighted, parallel to the sacrum
(plot on mediosagittal slice), *fat-saturated*

> **Example**
> *TSE, FS:*
> — TR = 2500–3500
> — TE = 80–120

or

TIRM or STIR

> **Example**
> *1.5 and 1.0 T:*   *0.5 T:*
> — TR = 6500   — TR = 2500
> — TE = 14   — TE = 60
> — TI = 140   — TI = 100
> — Flip angle 180°

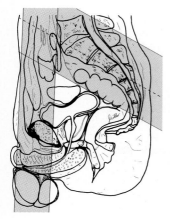

Sacroiliac joints, para-axial to the sacrum, sequence 2

- Slice thickness: 4–5 mm
- Slice gap: 10–20% of slice thickness ($\triangleq$ 0.4–1.0 mm or factor 1.1–1.2)
- FOV: medium, e.g., 250 mm
- Phase encoding gradient: AP (or HF, depending on the obliqueness) with 50% oversampling
- Matrix: 512, if possible
- Saturation slab: superior to the slices

Sequence 3 para-axial (as sequence 2)

T1-weighted

> **Example**
> *TSE:*
> - TR = 450–600
> - TE = 12–25

- Slice thickness: 4 mm
- Slice gap: 10–20% of slice thickness ($\triangleq$ 0.4–0.8 mm or factor 1.1–1.2)
- Phase encoding gradient: AP with 50% oversampling
- Saturation slab: superior to the slices

Sequence 4 paracoronal

T1-weighted

> **Example**
> *SE:*
> - TR = 500–700
> - TE = 12–25
> - Flip angle 90° or 150°

or

T2-weighted, TIRM or SPIR

> **Example**
> - TR = 6500   - TI = 140
> - TE = 14   - Flip angle 180°

or

T2-weighted, fat-saturated

> **Example**
> *TSE, FS:*
> — TR = 2500–3500
> — TE = 80–120

— Slice thickness: 4–6 mm
— Slice gap: 30–50% of slice thickness (≙ 1.2–3 mm or factor 1.3–1.5)
— Phase encoding gradient: AP
— Two saturation slabs:
  - Orthogonal (coronal) to the slices, ventral to the fatty tissue of the abdominal wall
  - Axial, superior to the slices, for saturation of the vessels

and possibly

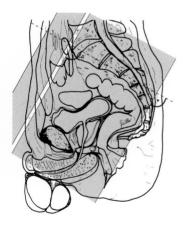

Sacroiliac joints, paracoronal, orthogonal to the sacrum, sequence 4

Sequence 5 paracoronal

T1-weighted, fat-saturated as sequence 4 but after administration of contrast agent (e.g., Gd-DTPA) (for visible pathology or investigation for infection, tumor, etc.)

Magnetic Resonance Angiography

Cervical Vessels

Patient Preparation
— Have the patient go to the toilet before the study
— Explain the procedure to the patient
— Ask the patient to undress except for underwear
— Ask the patient to remove anything containing metal (hearing aids, hairpins, body jewelry, etc.)
— Have a large-gauge intravenous line inserted with flushed extension set connected

Positioning
— Supine
— Neck coil (body array coil)
— Cushion the knees
— If necessary, offer the patient ear protectors

Sequences
— Scout: axial, sagittal, and coronal

If a test bolus is being used then either use a coronal slice as the plane for the test bolus or

Sequence 1 axial (test bolus)

T1-weighted across the center of the neck, GRE (total acquisition time per slice is 1 second; 30 slices in series in the same slice position)

Example
— TR = 5–8.5
— TE = 3–4.0
— Flip angle 10–40°

Start sequence simultaneously with the injection of 2 ml contrast (preinjected into the line and followed by 20 ml saline; e.g., Gd-BOPTA or gadobutrol

Injection rate:
Bolus injection (approx. 2–3 ml/s). Determine the time required from the start of the injection until maximum signal (e.g., in carotid artery) is reached (= "contrast circulation time"); divide the total duration of the angiography sequence (= sequence 2 below) by 2 and subtract the contrast circulation time from this result. This yields the time in seconds needed to start the contrast injection ahead of (for negative values) or after (for positive values) the start of the sequence.

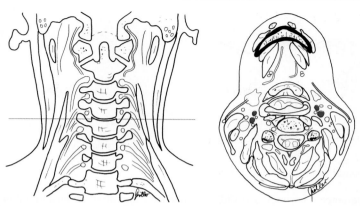

Cervical vessels, axial, test bolus, sequence 1

Sequence 2 coronal, 3-D GRE noncontrast (e.g., FISP)

> **Example**
> — TR = 6.8
> — TE = 2.3
> — Flip angle 45°
> *3-D FFE:*
> — TR = 2.5–5
> — TE = 1–2
> — Flip angle 25–40°

— Slab thickness: 50–60 mm
— No. of partitions: 28–36
— FOV: large (400 mm)
— Matrix 512 (256)

The injection of the contrast agent depends on the duration of the sequence (e.g., 30 seconds) and the contrast circulation time (measured) (e.g., 12 seconds). The contrast peak must be in the center of the k-space = usually in the middle of the sequence (in our case = 30/2=15 seconds; since the contrast agent will start flooding after 12 seconds, contrast injection will have to begin 3 seconds after the start of the sequence).

Injection rate: 1–2 ml/s

Amount of contrast agent needed: 20 (–40) ml of, e.g., Gd-BOPTA or 10–20 ml gadobutrol

Sequence 3 coronal, 3-D GRE, as sequence 2, but after administration of contrast agent

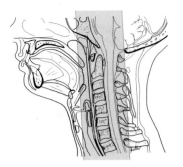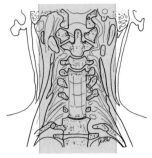

Cervical vessels, sequence 2 coronal

Sequence 4 coronal, 3-D GRE, as sequence 2, but after administration of contrast agent

Postprocessing
— Subtraction: sequence 3 minus sequence 2 and sequence 4 minus sequence 2
— MIP analysis

Tips & Tricks
— Have the patient swallow before the study
  Note: ask the patient not to swallow during the study
— A second scout in the form of a short sagittal phase contrast series (e.g., 1.5 T: TR = 81, TE = 9, flip angle = 11°, thickness = 60 mm, flow 45–45–45) across one side may improve adjustment. This has the advantage of allowing direct adjustment over the vessels and allowing a smaller slab to be used
— *Note:* some companies use sequences where the center of the *k*-space does not coincide with the middle of the acquisition period; check with the company and adjust the timing accordingly
— The rule of thumb for the injection rate is:
  Volume of injection/half the duration of the sequence = injection rate in ml/s
— For the test bolus it may be better to select the beginning or middle of the rise in signal intensity after contrast injection and not the maximum contrast signal as test bolus time (contrast circulation time); this places the bolus tighter around the center of the *k*-space. The aim is to avoid the venous contrast phase
— With manual contrast injection an additional 1–2 seconds may be needed to compensate for the reaction time

Thoracic Aorta

Patient Preparation
— Have the patient go to the toilet before the study
— Explain the procedure to the patient
— Ask the patient to undress except for underwear
— Ask the patient to remove anything containing metal (hearing aids, hairpins, body jewelry, etc.)
— Have a large-gauge intravenous line inserted and flushed extension set connected

Positioning
— Supine
— Body coil (or body array coil)
— Cushion the knees
— If necessary, offer the patient ear protectors

Sequences
— Scout: axial, sagittal, and coronal

If a test bolus is being used then either paracoronal slice or

Sequence 1 axial

T1-weighted across the aorta, GRE (total acquisition time per slice is 1 second; 30 slices in series in the same slice position)

Example
— TR = 5–8.5
— TE = 3–4.0
— Flip angle 10–40°

Start sequence simultaneously with the injection of 2 ml contrast (preinjected into the line and followed by 20 ml saline; e.g., Gd-BOPTA or gadobutrol)

Injection rate: Bolus injection (approx. 2–3 ml/s)
Determine the time required from the start of the injection until maximum signal in the thoracic aorta is reached (= contrast circulation time); divide the total duration of the angiography sequence (= sequence 2 below) by 2 and subtract the time to maximum signal (contrast circulation time) from this result. This yields the time in seconds needed to start the contrast injection ahead of (for negative values) or after (for positive values) the start of the sequence.

Injection of the contrast agent depends on the duration of the sequence (e.g., 34 seconds) and the contrast circulation time (measured) (e.g., 10 seconds). The contrast peak must be in the center of the *k*-space = usually in the middle of the sequence (in our case = 34/2=17 seconds; since the contrast agent will start flooding after 10 seconds, contrast injection will have to begin 7 seconds before the start of the sequence).

Injection rate: 1.5–2.5 ml/s
Amount of contrast agent needed: 20 (–40) ml of, e.g., Gd-BOPTA or 10–20 ml gadobutrol

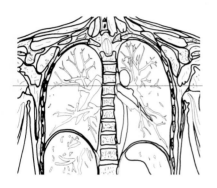

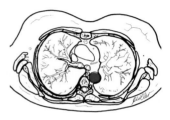

Thoracic aorta, axial, test bolus, sequence 1

Sequence 2 (para-) coronal, 3-D GRE breathhold (e.g., in inspiration) with contrast enhancement (e.g., FISP)

Example
— TR = 5.8
— TE = 1.8
— Flip angle 30°
3-D FFE:
— TR = 2.5–5
— TE = 1–2
— Flip angle 25–40°

— Slab thickness: 60–80 mm
— No. of partitions: 28–36
— FOV: large (500 mm)
— Matrix: 512 (256)

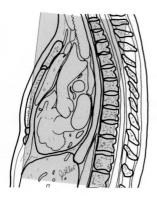
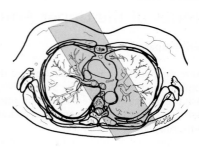

Thoracic aorta, coronal,
sequence 2

Possibly after another respiration cycle
(delay to start of sequence 3 approx. 5–7 seconds)

Sequence 3 coronal as sequence 2, but after contrast enhancement (late image)

Postprocessing
— MIP analysis

Tips & Tricks
- *Note:* use a large-gauge intravenous line
- *Note:* some companies use sequences where the center of the k-space does not coincide with the middle of the acquisition period; check with the company and adjust the timing accordingly
- The rule of thumb for the injection rate is:
  Volume of injection/half the duration of the sequence = injection rate in ml/s
- With manual contrast injection an additional 3 seconds may be needed to compensate for the reaction time

---

Arteries of the Upper Arm

Patient Preparation

— Have the patient go to the toilet before the study
— Explain the procedure to the patient
— Ask the patient to undress except for underwear
— Ask the patient to remove anything containing metal (hearing aids, hairpins, rings, body jewelry, etc.)
— Insert large-gauge intravenous line in other arm and connect flushed extension set

Positioning
— Supine
— Body coil (or body array coil)
— Cushion the knees
— If necessary, offer the patient ear protectors

Sequences
— Scout: axial, sagittal, and coronal
  If a test bolus is being used then

Sequence 1 axial

T1-weighted across the upper arm, GRE (total acquisition time per slice is 1 second; 30 slices in series in the same slice position)

Example
— TR = 5–8.5
— TE = 3–4.0
— Flip angle 10–40°

Start sequence simultaneously with the injection of 2 ml contrast (preinjected into the line and followed by 20 ml saline; e.g., Gd-BOPTA)

Injection rate: Bolus injection (approx. 2–3 ml/s)
Determine the time required from the start of the injection until maximum signal in the brachial artery is reached (= contrast circulation time); divide the total duration of the angiography sequence (= sequence 2 below) by 2 and subtract the time to maximum signal (contrast circulation time) from this result. This yields the time in seconds needed to start the contrast injection ahead of (for negative values) or after (for positive values) the start of the sequence.

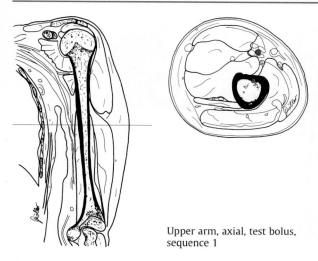

Upper arm, axial, test bolus,
sequence 1

Sequence 2 coronal, 3-D GRE breathhold (e.g., in inspiration), noncontrast
(e.g., FISP)

Example
— TR = 6.8
— TE = 2.3
— Flip angle 45°
3-D FFE:
— TR = 2.5–5
— TE = 1–2
— Flip angle 25–40°

— Slab thickness: 50–70 mm
— No. of partitions: 25–35
— FOV: large (500 mm)
— Matrix: 512 (256)

Injection of the contrast agent depends on the duration of the sequence (e.g.,
30 seconds) and the contrast circulation time measured (e.g., 10 seconds).
The contrast peak must be in the center of the k-space = usually in the
middle of the sequence (in our case = 30/2=15 seconds; since the contrast
agent will start flooding after 10 seconds, contrast injection will have to
begin 5 seconds after the start of the sequence).

Injection rate: 1–2 ml/s
Amount of contrast agent needed: 20 (–40) ml of, e.g., Gd-BOPTA

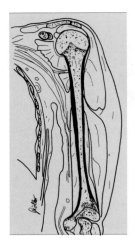
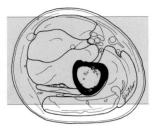

Upper arm, coronal,
sequence 2

After another respiration cycle
(delay to start of sequence 3 approx. 5–7 seconds)

Sequence 3 coronal as sequence 2, but after contrast enhancement

Sequence 4 coronal (if the scanner allows) as sequence 3 after another respiration cycle (approx. 5–7 seconds)

Postprocessing
— MIP analysis after the subtraction (sequences 3 and 4 minus sequence 2)

Tips & Tricks
  — *Note:* use a large-gauge intravenous line
  — *Note:* some companies use sequences where the center of the k-space does not coincide with the middle of the acquisition period; check with the company and adjust the timing accordingly
  — The rule of thumb for the injection rate is:
    Volume of injection/half the duration of the sequence = injection rate in ml/s
  — With manual contrast injection an additional 3 seconds may be needed to compensate for the reaction time

Arteries of the Forearm

Patient Preparation
— Have the patient go to the toilet before the study
— Explain the procedure to the patient
— Ask the patient to undress except for underwear
— Ask the patient to remove anything containing metal (hearing aids, hairpins, rings, body jewelry, etc.)
— Have intravenous line inserted in other arm with flushed extension set connected

Positioning
— Supine (possibly prone)
— Body array coil or surface coil (possibly body coil)
— If necessary, offer the patient ear protectors

Sequences
— Scout: axial, sagittal, and coronal

   If a test bolus is being used then

Sequence 1 axial

T1-weighted across the distal upper arm or proximal forearm, GRE (total acquisition time per slice is 1 second; 30 slices in series in the same slice position)

Example
— TR = 5–8.5
— TE = 3–4.0
— Flip angle 10–40°

Start sequence simultaneously with the injection of 2 ml contrast (preinjected into the line and followed by 20 ml saline; e.g., Gd-BOPTA or gadobutrol)

Injection rate: Bolus injection (approx. 2–3 ml/s)
Determine the time required from the start of the injection until maximum signal in the brachial artery is reached (= contrast circulation time); divide the total duration of the angiography sequence (= sequence 2 below) by 2 and subtract the time to maximum signal (contrast circulation time) from this result. This yields the time in seconds needed to start the contrast injection ahead of (for negative values) or after (for positive values) the start of the sequence.

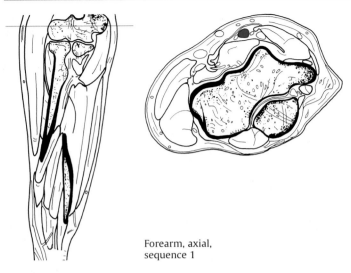

Forearm, axial,
sequence 1

Sequence 2 coronal, 3-D GRE noncontrast (e.g., FISP)

Example
— TR = 5.8
— TE = 1.8
— Flip angle 30°
3-D FFE:
— TR = 2.5–5
— TE = 1–2
— Flip angle 25–40°

— Slab thickness: 45–70 mm
— No. of partitions: 20–35
— FOV: large (400–500 mm)
— Matrix: 512 (256)

Injection of the contrast agent depends on the duration of the sequence (e.g., 30 seconds) and the contrast circulation time measured (e.g., 12 seconds). The contrast peak must be in the center of the k-space = usually in the middle of the sequence (in our case = 30/2=15 seconds; since the contrast agent will start flooding after 12 seconds, contrast injection will have to begin 3 seconds after the start of the sequence). [*Note:* since the test bolus is acquired across the proximal forearm, this is really about 2 seconds too early, because the contrast agent takes longer to reach the whole of the forearm. This can be compensated by increasing the duration of the injection, so it is better to select a slower injection rate, thus prolonging the injection.])

Injection rate: 1–2 ml/s
Amount of contrast agent: 20 (–40) ml, e.g., Gd-BOPTA or 10–20 ml gadobutrol

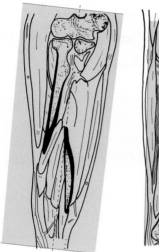 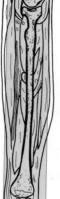 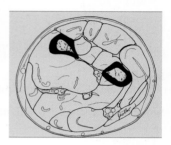

Forearm, coronal, sequence 2

Sequence 3 coronal as sequence 2, but after contrast enhancement
Sequence 4 coronal (if the scanner allows) as sequence 3

Postprocessing
— MIP analysis after the subtraction (sequences 3 and 4 minus sequence 2)

Tips & Tricks
— *Note:* some companies use sequences where the center of the *k*-space does not coincide with the middle of the acquisition period; check with the company and adjust the timing accordingly
— The rule of thumb for the injection rate is:
  Volume of injection/half the duration of the sequence = injection rate in ml/s
— With manual contrast injection an additional 3 seconds may be needed to compensate for the reaction time

Arteries of the Hand

Patient Preparation
— Have the patient go to the toilet before the study
— Explain the procedure to the patient
— Ask the patient to undress except for underwear
— Ask the patient to remove anything containing metal (hearing aids, hairpins, body jewelry, etc.)
— Have intravenous line inserted in other arm with flushed extension set connected
— Rest the hand to be studied in a bowl of warm water
— Keep nitroglycerin spray ready

Positioning
— Supine or prone
— Surface coil
— If the supine position is adopted, it may be helpful to use a hand rest

Sequences
— Scout: axial, sagittal, and coronal

Sequence 1 coronal, 3-D GRE noncontrast (e.g., FISP)

Example
— TR = 5.8
— TE = 1.8
— Flip angle 30°
3-D FFE:
— TR = 2.5–5
— TE = 1–2
— Flip angle 25–40°

— Slab thickness: 40–50 mm
— No. of partitions: 15–25
— FOV: medium (250–350 mm)
— Matrix: 512 (256)

Injection of the contrast agent depends on the duration of the sequence (e.g., 18 seconds) and the contrast circulation time measured (e.g., 15 seconds). The contrast peak must be in the center of the k-space = usually in the middle of the sequence (for the hand it could be selected such that the contrast agent starts arriving about one-quarter of the contrast circulation time after acquisition begins).

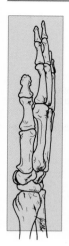 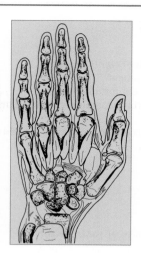

Hand, coronal, sequence 1

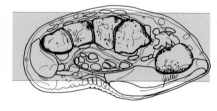

Injection rate: 1–2 ml/s
(Select a rate such that the injection takes approximately two-thirds of the acquisition time)
Amount of contrast agent: 20 (–40) ml of, e.g., Gd-BOPTA or 10–20 ml gadobutrol

Sequences 2–6 coronal as sequence 1 but after administration of contrast agent

Postprocessing
— MIP analysis after the subtraction (sequences 2–6 minus sequence 1)

Tips & Tricks
— 1–2 sprays of nitroglycerin may be given before the study

Abdominal Aorta

Patient Preparation
— Have the patient go to the toilet before the study
— Explain the procedure to the patient
— Ask the patient to undress except for underwear
— Ask the patient to remove anything containing metal (hearing aids, hairpins, body jewelry, etc.)
— Have a large-gauge intravenous line inserted with flushed extension set connected

Positioning
— Supine
— Body coil
— Cushion the knees
— If necessary, offer the patient wear ear protectors

Sequences
— Scout: axial, sagittal, and coronal

If a test bolus is being used then either coronal or

Sequence 1 axial

T1-weighted across the aorta, GRE (total time of acquisition per slice is 1 second; 30 slices in series in the same slice position)

Example
TSE:
— TR = 5–8.5
— TE = 3–4.0
— Flip angle 10–40°

Start sequence simultaneously with the injection of 2 ml contrast (preinjected into the line and followed by 20 ml saline; e.g., Gd-BOPTA or gadobutrol.

Injection rate: Bolus injection (approx. 2–3 ml/s)
Determine the time required from the start of the injection until maximum signal in the abdominal aorta is reached (= contrast circulation time); divide the total duration of the angiography sequence (= sequence 2 below) by 2 and subtract the time to maximum signal (contrast circulation time) from this result. This yields the time in seconds needed to start the contrast injection ahead of (for negative values) or after (for positive values) the start of the sequence.
Injection of the contrast agent depends on the duration of the sequence (e.g.,

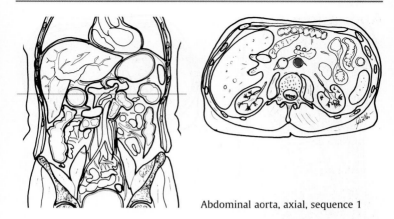

Abdominal aorta, axial, sequence 1

34 seconds) and the measured contrast circulation time (e.g., 13 seconds). The contrast peak must be in the center of the k-space = usually in the middle of the sequence (in our case = 34/2=17 seconds; since the contrast agent will start flooding after 13 seconds, contrast injection will have to begin 4 seconds after the start of the sequence).

Injection rate: 1.5–2.5 ml/s
Amount of contrast agent needed: 20 (–40) ml of, e.g., Gd-BOPTA or 10–20 ml gadobutrol

Sequence 2 coronal, 3-D GRE breathhold (e.g., in inspiration) after contrast enhancement (e.g., FISP)

Example
— TR = 5.8
— TE = 1.8
— Flip angle 30°
3-D FFE:
— TR = 2.5–6
— TE = 1–2
— Flip angle 25–40°

— Slab thickness: 60–80 mm
— No. of partitions: 28–36
— FOV: large (500 mm)
— Matrix: 512 (256)

Possibly after another respiration cycle

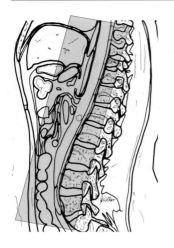
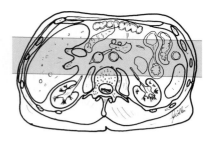

Abdominal aorta, coronal, sequence 2

(delay to start of sequence 3 approx. 5–7 seconds)

Sequence 3 coronal, 3-D GRE breathhold (e.g., in inspiration) after contrast enhancement (as sequence 2)

Postprocessing
— MIP analysis

Tips & Tricks
— Hyoscine butylbromide may be given intravenously to attenuate intestinal motility
— A strap across the abdomen will attenuate breathing motion and intestinal motility
— *Note:* use a large-gauge intravenous line
— *Note:* some companies use sequences where the center of the *k*-space does not coincide with the middle of the acquisition period; check with the company and adjust the timing accordingly
— The rule of thumb for the injection rate is:
  Volume of injection/half the duration of the sequence = injection rate in ml/s

Renal Arteries

Patient Preparation
— Have the patient go to the toilet before the study
— Explain the procedure to the patient
— Ask the patient to undress except for underwear
— Ask the patient to remove anything containing metal (hearing aids, hair-pins, rings, body jewelry, etc.)
— Have a large-gauge intravenous line placed with flushed extension set connected

Positioning
— Supine
— Body coil (body array coil)
— Cushion the knees
— If necessary, offer the patient wear ear protectors

Sequences
— Scout: axial, sagittal, and coronal

If a test bolus is being used then either coronal or

Sequence 1 axial

T1-weighted across the aortic origin of the renal arteries, GRE (total acquisition time per slice is 1 second; 30 slices in series in the same slice position)

Example
TSE:
— TR = 5–8.5
— TE = 3–4.0
— Flip angle 10–40°

Start sequence simultaneously with the injection of 2 ml contrast (preinjected into the line and followed by 20 ml saline; e.g., Gd-BOPTA or gadobutrol).

Injection rate: Bolus injection (approx. 2–3 ml/s)
Determine the time required from the start of the injection until maximum signal in the abdominal aorta is reached (= contrast circulation time); divide the total duration of the angiography sequence (= sequence 2 below) by 2 and subtract the time to maximum signal (contrast circulation time) from this result. This yields the time in seconds needed to start the contrast injection ahead of (for negative values) or after (for positive values) the start of the sequence.

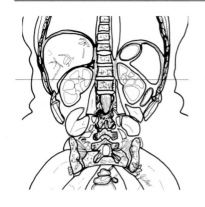
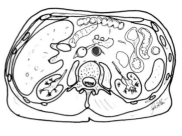

Renal arteries, axial, test bolus, sequence 1

Injection of the contrast agent depends on the duration of the sequence (e.g., 34 seconds) and the measured contrast circulation time (e.g., 13 seconds). The contrast peak must be in the center of the k-space = usually in the middle of the sequence (in our case = 34/2=17 seconds; since the contrast agent will start flooding after 13 seconds, contrast injection will have to begin 4 seconds after the start of the sequence).

Injection rate: 1.5–2.5 ml/s
Amount of contrast agent needed: 20 (–40) ml of, e.g., Gd-BOPTA or 10–20 ml gadobutrol

Sequence 2 coronal, 3-D GRE breathhold (e.g., in inspiration) with contrast enhancement (e.g., FISP)

Example
Example
— TR = 5.8
— TE = 1.8
— Flip angle 30°
3-D FFE:
— TR = 2.5–5
— TE = 1–2
— Flip angle 25–40°

— Slab thickness: 60–80 mm
— No. of partitions: 28–36
— FOV: large (500 mm)
— Matrix: 512 (256)

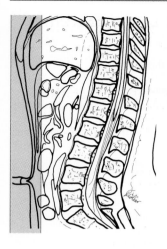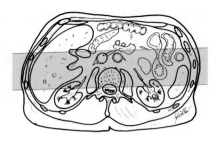

Renal arteries, coronal, sequence 2

**Perhaps after another respiration cycle
(delay to start of sequence 3 approx. 5–7 seconds)**

**Sequence 3 coronal, 3-D GRE breathhold (e.g., in inspiration), but after
contrast enhancement** (as sequence 2)

Postprocessing
— MIP analysis

Tips & Tricks
— Hyoscine butylbromide may be given intravenously to attenuate in-
  testinal motility
— A strap across the lower abdomen will attenuate breathing motion and
  intestinal motility
— *Note:* Use a large-gauge intravenous line
— *Note:* Some companies use sequences where the center of the *k*-space
  does not coincide with the middle of the acquisition period; check with
  the company and adjust the timing accordingly
— The rule of thumb for the injection rate is:
  Volume of injection/half the duration of the sequence = injection rate
  in ml/s

Arteries of the Pelvis and Lower Extremity

Patient Preparation
— Have the patient go to the toilet before the study
— Explain the procedure to the patient
— Ask the patient to undress except for underwear
— Ask the patient to remove anything containing metal (hearing aids, hair-pins, rings, body jewelry, etc.)
— Have a large-gauge intravenous line placed with flushed extension set connected

Positioning
— Supine
— Body coil (body array coil)
— Cushion the legs such that ankle and hip are level
— If necessary offer the patient ear protectors
— Secure the legs (sandbags, straps, vacuum mattress)

Double-Bolus Technique

Sequences
— Scout: axial, sagittal, and coronal

Lower Leg

If a test bolus is being used then

Sequence 1 axial

T1-weighted across the popliteal artery (total acquisition time per slice is 2 seconds; 30 slices in series in the same slice position or 60 slices at 1 second each)

Example
TSE:
— TR = 5–8.5
— TE = 3–4.0
— Flip angle 10–40°

Start sequence simultaneously with the injection of 2 ml contrast (preinjected into the line and followed by 20 ml saline; e.g., Gd-BOPTA or 1–2 ml gadobutrol).

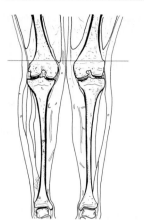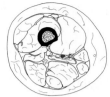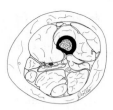

Arteries of the pelvis and lower extremity, axial, test bolus, sequence 1

Injection rate: Bolus injection (approx. 2–3 ml/s)

Determine the time required from the start of the injection until maximum signal in the popliteal artery is reached (= contrast circulation time); divide the total duration of the angiography sequence (= sequence 2 below) by 2 and subtract the time to maximum signal (contrast circulation time) from this result. This yields the time in seconds needed to start the contrast injection ahead of (for negative values) or after (for positive values) the start of the sequence.

Sequence 2 coronal, 3-D GRE noncontrast (e.g., FISP)

Example
— TR = 5.8
— TE = 1.8
— Flip angle 30°
3-D FFE:
— TR = 2.5–5
— TE = 1–2
— Flip angle 25–40°

— Slab thickness: 60–80 mm
— No. of partitions: 28–36
— FOV: large (500 mm)
— Matrix: 512 (256)

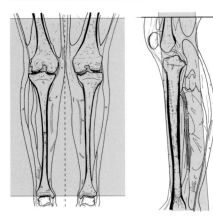

Arteries of the pelvis and lower extremity, coronal, sequence 2

Injection of the contrast agent depends on the duration of the sequence (e.g., 30 seconds) and the measured contrast circulation time (e.g., 17 seconds). The contrast peak must be in the center of the k-space = usually in the middle of the sequence (in our case = 30/2=15 seconds; since the contrast agent will start flooding after 17 seconds, contrast injection will have to begin 2 seconds before the start of the sequence).

Injection rate: 1–2 ml/s
Amount of contrast agent needed: 18–20 ml of, e.g., Gd-BOPTA or 10 ml of gadobutrol

Sequence 3 coronal, 3-D GRE, as sequence 2, but after administration of contrast agent

Sequence 4 coronal, 3-D GRE, as sequence 2, but after administration of contrast agent (late phase)

Iliofemoral Region

Sequence 5 coronal, 3-D GRE noncontrast (e.g., FISP)

Example	
— TR = 5.8	*3-D FFE:*
— TE = 1.8	— TR = 2.5–5
— Flip angle 30°	— TE = 1–2
	— Flip angle 25–40°

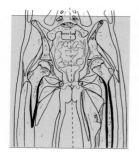 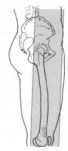 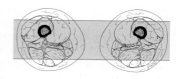

Iliofemoral region, coronal, sequence 5

— Slab thickness: 60–80 mm
— No. of partitions: 28–36
— FOV: large (500 mm)
— Matrix: 512 (256)

Sequence 6 coronal, 3-D GRE, as sequence 2, but after administration of contrast agent
Injection of the contrast agent depends on the duration of the sequence (e.g., 30 seconds) and the contrast circulation time (which may be estimated now: about 3–4 seconds less than the time measured for the lower leg, i.e., approx. 13–14 seconds. The contrast peak must be in the middle of the sequence (see above; in our case = 30/2=15 seconds; since the contrast agent will start flooding after [an estimated] 14 seconds, contrast injection will have to begin 1 second after the start of the sequence).

Injection rate: 1–2 ml/s
Amount of contrast agent: 20 ml of, e.g., Gd-BOPTA or 10 ml of gadobutrol

Sequence 7 coronal, 3-D GRE, as sequence 2, but after administration of contrast agent (late phase)

Postprocessing
— Subtraction: sequence 3 minus sequence 2 and sequence 6 minus sequence 5
— MIP analysis

Tips & Tricks
— Hyoscine butylbromide may be given intravenously to attenuate intestinal motility
— A strap across the lower abdomen will attenuate breathing motion and intestinal motility
— *Note:* use a large-gauge intravenous line

— Secure legs well (because of the subtraction)
— Elevate distal part of the legs somewhat and cushion well
— Have the patient move well into the scanner
— Perform MIP analysis of the late phases (sequence 4 minus sequence 2 and sequence 7 minus sequence 5) if the arteries of either or both legs are not yet visualized (e.g., arterial occlusion)
— *Note:* some companies use sequences where the center of the *k*-space does not coincide with the middle of the acquisition period; check with the company and adjust the timing accordingly
— The rule of thumb for the injection rate is:
Volume of injection/half the duration of the sequence = injection rate in ml/s
— With manual contrast injection, an additional 3–5 seconds may be needed to compensate for the reaction time

Modifications

Table Travel

Sequence 1 coronal, 3-D GRE noncontrast

> **Example**
> FFE:
> — TR = 8 (10)
> — TE = 2 (3)
> — Flip angle 30° (45°)

— Slice thickness: 1.25–1.5 mm (3 mm for 0.5 T)
— No. of slices: 60–80 (25 for 0.5 T)
— FOV: large (450 mm)
— Matrix: 512 (256 for 0.5 T)
— Phase encoding gradient: RL
— Three stations:
   • Start the sequences by setting up the masks (beginning with the lower leg and ending with the pelvis)
   • Contrast injection: 0.3–0.6 ml/s (split into two bolus phases: volume 1 = 20 ml, flow rate: 0.6 ml/s; volume 2 = 18 ml, flow rate: 0.3 ml/s); amount of contrast agent: 30–50 ml Gd-BOPTA
   • After about 40 seconds start the angiography sequence (begin with the iliac region) with three regions

References

Aschoff, A. J., H. Zeitler, E. M. Merkle, M. Reishagen, H.-J. Brambs, A. Rieber: MR-Enteroklyse zur kernspintomographischen Diagnostik entzündlicher Darmerkrankungen mit verbesserter Armkontrastierung. Fortschr. Röntgenstr 167 (1997)

Bundesausschuss der Ärzte und Krankenkassen: Richtlinien über Kriterien zur Qualitätsbeurteilung in der Kernspintomographie. Dtsch. Ärztebl. 98 (2001)

Dong, Q., S. O. Schoenberg, R. C. Carlos et al.: Diagnosis of renal vascular disease with MR angiography. Radiographics 19 (1999) 1535

Elster, A. D.: Modern imaging of the pituitary. Radiology 187 (1993) 1

Gaa, J., K.-J. Lehmann, M. Georgi: MRAngiographie und Elektronenstrahl-CT-Angiographie. Thieme, Stuttgart 2000

Hamm, B., G. P. Krestin, M. Laniado, V. Nicolas: MRT von Abdomen und Becken. Thieme, Stuttgart 1999

Heindel, W., H. Kugel, K. Lackner: Rationelle MR-Untersuchungstechniken. Thieme, Stuttgart 1997

Helmberger, H., K. Hellerhoff, Th. Rüll, Ch. Brandt, P. Gerhardt: Funktionelle MR-Pankreatikographie mit Sekretin. Fortschr. Röntgenstr. 172 (2000) 367

Holzknecht, N., T. Helmberger, C. von Ritter, J. Gauger, S. Faber, M. Reiser: Dünndarm-MRT mit schnellen MR-Sequenzen bei Morbus Crohn nach Enteroklysma mit oralen Eisenpartikeln. Radiologe 38 (1998)

Krestin, G. P.: Morphologic and Functional MR of the Kidneys and Adrenal Glands. Fields & Wood, New York 1991

Lenhart, M., B. Djavidani, M. Völk et al.: Kontrastmittelverstärkte MR-Angiographie der Becken-Beingefäße mit automatisierter Tischverschiebetechnik. Fortschr. Röntgenstr. 171 (1999) 442

Mäurer, J., J. Rudolph, M. Lorang et al.: ProspektiveStudie zum Nachweis von Läsionen des Labrum glenoidale mit der indirekten MR-Arthrographie der Schulter. Fortschr. Röntgenstr. 171 (1999) 307

Möller, T. B., E. Reif: Taschenatlas Einstelltechnik. Thieme, Stuttgart 2000

Möller, T. B., E. Reif: Rezeptbuch radiologischer Verfahren. Springer, Heidelberg 2001

Munk, P. L., C. A. Helms: MRI of the Knee. Lippincott-Raven, Philadelphia 1996

Obenauer, S., U. Fischer, M. Heuser, R. Wilke, E. Grabbe: Optimierung der MR-Cholangiopankreatikographie. Fortschr. Röntgenstr. 171 (1999) 450

Seitz, J., P. Held, A. Waldeck, M. Völk, M. Lenhart, M. Strotzer: 3D CISS, 3D MPRAGE und 2DTSE für die präoperative MRT vor Cochlea Implant. Fortschr. Röntgenstr. 172 (2000) 227

Schunk, K., A. Kern, C. P. Heußel et al.: Hydro-MRT mit schnellen Sequenzen bei Morbus Crohn: Vergleich mit der fraktionierten Magen-Darm-Passage. Fortschr. Röntgenstr. 170 (1999)

Stark, D. D., W. G. Bradley Jr.: Magnet Resonance Imaging. Mosby, St. Louis 1999

Stoller, D. W.: MRI in Orthopaedics & Sports Medicine. Lippincott-Raven, Philadelphia 1997

Vahlensieck, M., M. Reiser: MRT des Bewegungsapparats. Thieme, Stuttgart 1997

Vitellas, K.M., M. T. Keogan, Ch. E. Spritzer, R. C. Nelson: MR cholangiopancreaticography of bile and pancreatic duct abnormalities with emphasis on the single-shot fast spin-echo technique. Radiographics 20 (2000) 939

Wintersperger, B. J., A.Huber,G. Preissler et al.: MR-Angiographie der supraaortalenGefäße. Radiologe 40 (2000) 785

Glossary

Acquisition time	Period of time required to collect the image data
AP	Anteroposterior = from the front to the back of the body
Axial	Orthogonal to the long axis of the body
CISS	Constructive interference steady state: a sequence which supposedly minimizes the interference-induced artifacts of a true FISP sequence; the CISS sequence is heavily T2-weighted and currently is used primarily as a high-resolution 3-D sequence for the inner ear
Coil	Transmission or reception unit for the signals transmitted/received by the magnet. There are transmission, reception, and combined transmission/reception coils, and they come as body and surface coils, the latter being available as rigid and flexible (wraparound) coils
Coronal	Frontal: a plane made by cutting across the body from side to side (left to right or right to left)
CSF	Cerebrospinal fluid
Dark fluid	Turbo inversion recovery sequence: a technique with a long TI (approx. 2200 ms for 1.0 and 1.5 T) used for fluid suppression, e.g., for suppressing the CSF in brain and spinal studies with T2 weighting (and long TE)
DESS	Dual echo steady state: gradient echo sequence where both axial and transverse magnetization adds to the signal, e.g. the FISP sequence and its temporally reversed form PSIF. In DESS the two sequences (FISP as a ratio of T1 to T2, and PSIF as mostly T2-weighted sequence) are added
3-D measurement	Volume measurement: imaging technique where each pulse excites not just a single slice but the entire volume of interest
Dual echo	Dual measurement: sequences characterized by two readout times (TE) for one (comparatively long) TR. Normally dual echo combines proton-density-weighted (short TE) and T2-weighted (long TE) measurements
ECG triggering (EGG gating)	Triggered by the signals of the heart: data acquisition takes place only during particular phases of the cardiac cycle (e.g. during systole or diastole); the patient has to be attached to a set of ECG leads

FFE	Fast field echo = FISP (fast imaging with steady state) = GRE (gradient echo) = GRASS (gradient recalled acquisition of steady state): gradient echo imaging where axial and transverse magnetization are combined and the contrast is the ratio of T1 to T2
FH	From feet to head
FISP	Fast imaging with steady state (see *FFE*)
FLAIR	Fluid attenuated inversion recovery (see *TIRM [dark fluid]*)
FLASH	Fast low angle shot = T1-weighted FFE = SPGR (spoiled GRASS): during steady state only the axial magnetization is used while the transverse magnetization is destroyed by „spoiling." Either T1- or T2-weighted contrast may be selected
Flip angle	= Pulse angle (PA): angle of excitation of the magnetization; for GRE sequences it is usually <90°; its value defines the degree of T1 weighting and thus must always be set for GRE sequences; normally for SE sequences the angle is 90°
Flow compensation	This technique avoids motion-induced signal loss and faulty acquisition
Foldover	Aliasing: artifact which mirrors (folds over) structures outside the sample field into the image; it arises in the direction of the phase-encoding gradient
FOV	Field of view: the slice region actually displayed
FS	Fat saturation (see *SPIR*)
FSE	Fast spin echo (see *TSE*)
Gadobutrol	Gadovist: a contrast agent based on gadolinium which is offered in a more concentrated form; particularly useful wherever a powerful bolus within a small volume is needed (e.g., in angiography)
Gd-BOPTA	Gadobenate dimeglumine; MultiHance
Gd-DTPA	Gadolinium diethylenetriamine pentaacetic acid complex, a gadolinium chelate; a contrast agent, such as Magnevist, which shortens T1 (positive action)
GRASS	Gradient-recalled acquisition of steady state (see *FFE*)
GRE	Gradient-recalled echo = gradient echo (see *FFE*)
HASTE sequence	Half-Fourier acquisition single-shot turbo spin echo: T2-weighted sequence where all of the image data is acquired in just one excitation pulse; characterized by short acquisition time per image and robustness to patient and respiration motion
HF	From head to feet

IR	Inversion recovery: a pulse sequence where the magnetization is inverted by a 180° pulse before the excitation pulses for signal acquisition are started. The period between the inversion pulse and the 90° pulse is called the inversion time (TI) and defines the degree of T1-weighting. May be employed for T1-weighted imaging as well as fat suppression (with short TI: STIR) or fluid suppression (with long TI: FLAIR, TIRM)
LR	Left to right
Lumirem	A suspension containing magnetite (iron): oral contrast agent making the intestines appear „dark"
Matrix	Image matrix: defines the number of pixels along each axis of the image, e.g., 128, 256, or 512 pixels
MIP	Maximum intensity projection: an image processing method where all high-intensity signals are filtered and projected in one plane
Midsagittal	The median plane of an object (in the anteroposterior direction)
Motion artifact suppression	A method of suppressing motion artifacts
MRA	Magnetic resonance angiography
MRI	Magnetic resonance imaging
NEX	Number of excitations (see *NSA*)
NSA	Number of signal averages = NEX (number of excitations) = how often a sequence is repeated; repetition improves the signal-to-noise ratio and thus image quality
Oral contrast agent	Used for contrast enhancement of the intestines
Orientation	Spatial arrangement of the slices
Oversampling	Foldover suppression: a method employed to avoid artifacts due to foldover
PA	Posteroanterior: from the back to the front of the body
Parasagittal	Plane through the body at an angle to the strict anteroposterior plane
Partition	Subdivision of a 3-D slab of data; the higher the number of partitions, the higher the resolution
Phase-encoding gradient	Foldover direction: there are foldover artifacts (aliasing) as well as pulsation artifacts along the direction of the phase-encoding gradient
Phase contrast angiography	The change in the phase shifts of the flowing protons in the region of interest are used to create an image

Proton-density-weighted	Pulse sequences with short TE and long TR, i.e., the images are neither T1- nor T2-weighted
PSIF	A sequence characterized by a heavily T2-weighted contrast with a short acquisition time; temporally reversed FISP sequence (from which it derives its name). FISP weighting is suppressed during steady-state acquisition. This sequence is sensitive to flow and motion artifacts
RARE	Refocused acquisition in readout direction
RES	Reticuloendothelial system of the liver, which takes up, e.g., ferruginous contrast agents
Respiration triggering	Data acquisition takes place only during one particular phase of the respiration cycle (e.g., inspiration or expiration). Usually the sensor is housed in a strap around the chest
RL	From right to left
Saturation	Spin excitation by means of, e.g., a rapid train of pulses such that the T1 relaxation is suppressed and the spins remain in the xy-plane in a dephased state. In successive pulse trains saturated pulses are not available for imaging and thus do not contribute to the image signal
Sagittal	Cross-section of the body in the anteroposterior plane
Scout	Planning scan = localizer= survey: a rapidly performed initial MR scan for orientation and planning purposes
SE	Spin echo: imaging where the spins used to generate the echo are refocused by a 180° pulse. Iin conventional pulsing one or more echoes with fixed phase encoding are read out for each excitation pulse
Sequence	This term denotes the set of imaging parameters in MRI, a „sequence" of specific excitations, pulse trains, and readout times
Signal-to-noise ratio	The ratio of the signal acquired to the background noise: the higher the number, the better the image
Single-slice technique	Only one slice is acquired but it is rather thick. The technique is only useful in fluid imaging (e.g., the biliary tree) where the surrounding tissue produces only a weak echo
Slab thickness	Thickness of a volume excited during 3-D imaging
Slice gap	The gap between two slices (1.1 = 10% gap; for a slice thickness of 8 mm this means a gap of 0.8 mm)

SNR	Signal-to-noise ratio
SPGR	Spoiled GRASS (see *FLASH*)
SPIR	Spectral presaturation with inversion recovery = frequency-selective fat suppression = FS: fat suppression where the fat signal is excited by frequency-selective saturation or inversion pulses such that it does not contribute anything to the image intensity
STIR	Short TI inversion recovery: inversion recovery pulse sequence with short TI for fat suppression. All signals with short T1 times similar to that of fat will be suppressed and usually they will not be displayed after contrast administration
Supermagnetic contrast agent	Contrast agent which shortens T2 (negative action): solid compounds which are administered as an oral suspension (unlike to the intravenous route of paramagnetic contrast agents) and become phagocytosed by the RES of the liver. For example, iron oxides with dextran coating (e.g., Endorem)
T1-FE	see *FLASH*
T1-weighted	Imaging with short repetition (TR) and echo time (TE). In T1-weighted images tissue with a short T1 is bright, while tissue with a long T1 is dark
T2-weighted	Imaging with long repetition (TR) and echo time (TE). In T2-weighted images tissue with a short T2 is dark, while tissue with a long T2 is bright
TE	Echo time: the time between the excitation and the middle of the readout process
TE shortest	The scanner automatically selects the shortest TE possible
Tesla	The unit of magnetic field strength (magnetic flux density). Named after Nikolaus Tesla, a nineteenth-century Croatian engineer. Abbreviated T
TF	Turbo factor
TI	Inversion time: in inversion recovery sequences, the time between the inversion pulse and the 90° pulse
TIRM (dark fluid)	Turbo inversion recovery measurement = (turbo) FLAIR = (turbo) inversion recovery
TOF	Time of flight: measurement method used in MR angiography. Unsaturated spins flow into a magnetized presaturated sample volume, and the differences between the unsaturated and presaturated spins are used to create the image

TR	Repetition time: the time between successive pulse sequences
TSE	Turbo spin echo = fast spin echo (FSE): fast spin echo measurement; multi-echo sequence within one TR period with varying phase encoding per echo
Turbo factor	The number of multiple echoes, and therefore the shortening of the measurement period compared to standard sequences

Appendix

Parameters for various field strengths

T1-weighted: The correlation between T1 and field strength is weak: TR for 1.5 T is the same as or slightly longer than TR for 0.5 T

TE: For the most part TE depends on the strength of the gradient. Most units with greater field strength also have a greater gradient strength. Thus, for example, TE (1.5 T): 12 ms; TE (1.0 T): 16 ms; TE (0.5 T): 24 ms.

T2-weighted: T2 is almost completely independent of the field strength. TR for 1.5 T corresponds to TR for 0.5 T.

Echo time in phase and out of phase: The echo times in phase and out of phase depend on the field strength:

1. Echo times in phase are even multiples and those out of phase (opposed-phase) are odd multiples of:
— 6.9 ms for 0.5 T
— 3.45 ms for 1.0 T
— 2.3 ms for 1.5 T

Phase-encoding gradient

Usually the phase-encoding gradient employed is:
— For sagittal images: PA
— For axial images: PA
— For coronal images: LR

Flip angle

For SE and TSE sequences the flip angle usually is 90° or 180°.

Slice sequence

Most often the slice sequence is set as interleaved, otherwise the slice gap is 1.2.

Scan parameters and their effects (based on Wolff)

Parameter	Resolution	Signal/noise ratio	Acquisition time	Remarks
FOV smaller	Better	Worse	No change	Overall fewer atoms contribute to the acquisition
Thinner slice	Better	Worse	No change	Overall fewer atoms contribute to the acquisition
Higher NSA	No change	Better	Longer	The signal is summed while some of the background noise is cancelled out
Scan % smaller	Worse	Better	Shorter	Since the acquisition field stays the same, pixel size and thus the number of atoms acquired must increase
Half-Scan	No change	Worse	Shorter	Fewer k-values

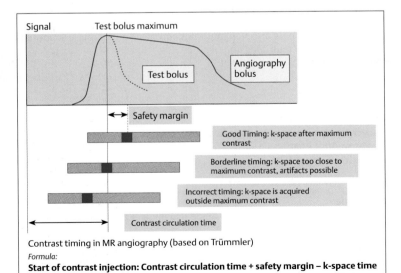

Contrast timing in MR angiography (based on Trümmler)

Formula:

Start of contrast injection: Contrast circulation time + safety margin – k-space time

k-Space time: usually half the duration of the sequence, although for some sequences it may be less, e. g., two-fifths of the duration of the sequence

Safety margin: usually between 1 and 5 seconds

Index